Health Policy in Europe:
Contemporary dilemmas and challenges

**Edited by Alexis Benos,
Hans Ulrich Deppe, John Lister**

International Association of Health Policy Europe (IAHPE)
www.healthp.org

Published by **International Association of Health Policy Europe** (IAHPE),
www.healthp.org

ISBN 978-0-9557333-0-7

Designed by John Lister, London Health Emergency,
www.healthemergency.org.uk
Cover painting: part of the work of Greek painter Nikos Anestis

Printed in Britain by Lightning Source UK Ltd

Introduction

Health policies in Europe from World War 2 up to the early 1980s were determined by the "welfarist consensus" and the dominance of Keynesianism (Lister, 2005) leading to the implementation of publicly funded and run health and social services. Standing in sharp contrast with the market-dominated reality of health and welfare in the USA, these policies established a European culture of social solidarity based on a wide range political consensus on the welfare state and redistributive economic measures.

However there were important differences between countries in the consistency of these policies, influenced by the variety of political and ideological background, which ranged from the pure social democratic tradition of the northern European countries to the liberal central Europe and the fascist dictatorships in the south (Portugal, Spain).

The neoliberal offensive that followed from the 1980s to the present day, and symbolically opened up by the Reagan and Thatcher administrations, established a new dominant ideology, one that:

> "assumes all governments, regardless of who governs, are forced to follow the same policies because of the need to be competitive in the globalised economy, where international markets determine what governments can and must do" (Navarro, 2002).

What governments must do – considered as "inevitable for the development" – is to open up their market and opportunities to make profits in all areas that had until the 1980s been considered to be of "public interest"– including energy, natural resources, transport, education, health and social services.

The European governments and the EU administration, unopposed by a labour movement which has itself remained in a deep ideological and political crisis, implemented neoliberal policies: these began with the dismantling, deregulation and often privatisation of public services, exposing them to market forces, imposing severe cutbacks in public expenditures and opening profit making opportunities for the private sector.

Disregarding the wealth of negative evidence coming from the American experiment in the dominance of private provision and the for profit market in health services, they are destroying the public sector, using as main ideological arguments the alleged 'efficiency', 'cost effectiveness' and 'quality' of services provided by the private sector – despite an absence of evidence to support these assumptions, and an abundance of evidence to the contrary. Defaming the public and community ethos and solidarity, they are promoting individualism, consumerism and civic passivity based on ignorance as the dominant values of the modern society.

One important aspect of this process driving the European societies backwards is that in several countries these policies have been promoted and implemented by social democratic forces with a long and dominant tradition in the labour movement. Nowadays the wide consensus between conservative and social democratic political forces in implementing neoliberal policies all over Europe gives definitive proof of the strategic crisis of social democracy, which despite the empty rhetoric of the so-called "third way" has proved itself to be ideologically and politically incapable of suggesting an alternative way forward. Nor do social democratic politicians understand the key lesson, that:

> "public services for health care and education provide the most obvious growing points for a new mode of production of value, not producing commodity values for the market, but use-values for the whole of society according to need" (J.T.Hart, 2006)..

This book is an effort to describe and critically analyse the recent experience of various European countries and discuss the dilemmas and challenges that confront health policy and policy-makers in this period of time and geopolitical setting, providing concrete evidence from various counties.

It is produced as an aftermath of the productive exchanges during the XIV Conference of the International Association of Health Policy in Europe (IAHPE), held in Thessaloniki in May 2005, through a peer review process. It is also an expression of the decision of IAHPE to enhance its main aim to promote critical analysis of the dominant health policies, both through conferences and published background material.

The first section of the book is an overview of contemporary policies in Europe and consists of chapters discussing their main characteristics under the dilemma 'Commercialisation or Solidarity'.

The second section consists of chapters presenting and critically analysing, aspects of the ongoing neoliberal reforms in several European countries from the north, west and south east European region.

In this section also, a paper published in *The International Journal of Health Services (IJHS)* presenting striking evidence from the US model of the potential consequences for European countries if the dominant ideological framework is allowed to continue to undermine universal and comprehensive health care services. This paper is reproduced with the permission of the *IJHS's* Editor, Vicente Navarro, a founding member of the International Association of Health Policy, whom we cordially thank for this contribution.

Alexis Benos, President

International Association of Health Policy in Europe (IAHPE)

References
John Lister (2005). *Health Policy Reform. Driving the wrong way? A Critical Guide to the Global "Health Reform" Industry.* Middlesex University Press.

Julia Tudor Hart, *The political economy of health care. A clinical perspective.* The Policy Press, University of Bristol.

Vicente Navarro (2002). *The political Economy of Social Inequalities. Consequences for Health and Quality of Life.* Baywood Publishing Company.

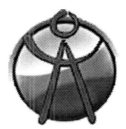

About IAHP

This volume has been produced by the International Association of Health Policy Europe, a regional organisation within the International Association of Health Policy (IAHP).

IAHP is a scientific, political and cultural organisation founded in 1977. It is an international network of scholars, health workers and activists with the aim of promoting the scientific analysis of public health issues and a forum for international comparisons and debate on health policy issues.

The basic principle adopted by IAHP members is the consideration of health as a social and political right. The main goal of the Association is the promotion of health, the struggle against health inequalities and the development of social solidarity.

The Association is interdisciplinary and gathers researchers from public health disciplines like social medicine, environmental and occupational health, epidemiology, medical sociology, health policy research, medical anthropology and health economics. A major subject is the interrelationship between theory and practice in health policy.

The main activity is regular conferences and seminars. These meetings cover a broad range of issues and they often gather both researchers and people involved in practical public health work and health policy. A major concern is also to develop the dialogue between North and South, East and West.

IAHP members in South America are active under the ALAMES and in Europe under the IAHP in Europe Association, which both have their own bodies and activities. There are members of IAHP all over the world working in various organisations and universities.

Contents

Section 1: OVERVIEW
Commercialisation or Solidarity?

Section 2:
COUNTRY STUDIES AND EXAMPLES

Commercialisation or Solidarity?
The Fundamental Orientation of Health Policy
Hans-Ulrich Deppe

In many areas of the public sector of our society, changes are taking place that utilize market economy instruments. This also applies to the delivery of health care; the basis of which, in the end, is determined by economic factors.

But where are the economic limitations? When do political or ethical questions become decisive for society?

The spreading, unreflected and uncontrolled application of economic laws and instruments onto non-economic circumstances and problems is described as 'economising'. This has correctly received the criticism, that individuals are thereby reduced to a 'homo economicus'. This does not constitute a general criticism on economics, but rather the denial of its omnipotence. The question is not just one of too strong an influence of economic principles, but whether the instruments which are being used are appropriate for the circumstances. Economics faces the danger of expanding beyond its limitations and becoming the standard of societal living, when it is allowed to dominate every aspect of society.

Under the hegemonic requirements of capital, markets and competition, society is reduced to a market society. Therefore, the question is which specific economic model forms the basis of the historically developed ruling structure?

Health or illness cannot entirely adopt the character of a marketable commodity. There is no health care system in the world that is organized solely on market-oriented principles. This is due, among other things, to the following peculiarities:

● With health, one is dealing with a good necessary for life. It is a collective and public good, similar to air, drinking water, education, traffic safety or legal security.

● One cannot, like other consumer goods, manage without health.

● The patient does not know when, or why s/he becomes sick, or which illness s/he will suffer from. S/he does not have the ability, to determine the appropriate extent, timing, or type of treatment. Illness is not something that can be managed by the individual, but is a general risk of life.

● The sovereignty of the consumer in the health care system is very limited.

● The demanding patient is confronted with the monopoly of medical knowledge, thereby creating supplier dominance.

● The demand of the patient as consumer is unspecific and is only defined and specified by the competence of a medical expert. There is an enormous information and competence asymmetry in favour of the doctor. The limited scientific nature of the practice of medicine allows considerable discretion in determining what diagnostic and therapeutic measures are undertaken.

● As a result of their illness, the patient is in a vulnerable position of uncertainty, weakness and dependency combined with fear and shame.

Describing the relationship between the market and the patient reveals the necessity for a public protection function. Much indicates that the delivery of health care is not amenable to the mechanisms of supply and demand.

The health care system is therefore an example of a failure of the market. The results that the distributive ability of the market could bring to bear are, in this case, insufficient. The market is a blind power. It must be given directions and objectives. The state, the democratic representation of society, therefore has important responsibilities and directional decisions must be made politically.

Within today's economic models, there are differences between a micro-economic and a macro-economic rationality. What is in the best interest of a business, is not necessarily sensible for the entire economy. Often the interests of the two dimensions are contradictory.

This is especially apparent in the case of environmental protection. The expansion of the micro-economic rationality today often means an enormous waste of societal resources. The company avoids the associated social costs, until society intervenes under macro-economic and social aspects. Even in the health care system this phenomenon can be observed, for example, in the shifting of costs from the ambulatory sector into the hospital sector: this can be advantageous for the individual institution, although it is more costly when viewed from a larger perspective.

As the Canadian health economist, Robert Evans, sarcastically but accurately remarks, from a micro-economic perspective, ineffective or even dangerous health care services can bring the same profits as effective and useful ones.(1)

Illness affects the intimate life of individuals

The primary place where illness is dealt with is in the intimacy of private life. The doctor-patient relationship(2) deals with specific social interactions that two individuals undertake outside of the public sphere of bourgeois society.

This intimate characteristic contradicts the necessary transparency of the market. At the same time we realize that the traditional roles within the individual spheres of society have changed since the beginning of the 1970s. That which was intimate has become more public. This is brought forward in questions of sexuality, psychiatric problems and the personal dismay of illness. One speaks of such things – openly. The self-help movement has also played an important role. A change in the doctor-patient relationship paralleled this development. In its original form it was paternal and authoritative, with the doctor acting as an agent for the immature patient.

The changes in this relationship have come slowly, and in a direction that is more partnership-oriented. This enables more patient participation and responsibility, and gives information and control increased importance. "The doctor as agent" becomes more and more "the doctor as trustee". (3)

The doctor-patient-relationship is asymmetrical

In medical sociology, the doctor-patient relationship remains asymmetrical. Differences in knowledge and instrumental capabilities, one-sided competence as well as sanctions and ordinances support the social position of the doctor with the power of an expert.

However, if and how the doctor uses this professional power, is dependent mostly on external influences. What role and priority professional power has in the decision on sources of income, what criteria are used to determine referrals and prescriptions, and what may be the formal and informal rules in the presentation of symptoms are therefore issues of importance.

In the ambulatory sector, competition has become an external factor not to be underestimated. It is well known, that the degree to which a doctor is "patient-centred" increases as competition for patients, and therefore income, increases. The adaptability of the contract doctor in Germany is limitless, whether this involves the location of their practice, their hours, the number of patients, what prescriptions they write, or what therapeutic measures they order, even if they are known to be ineffective – or even damaging.

Discretionary power, indications, and false diagnoses

Why do doctors have so many possibilities in their decision-making? It is not simply their being entrepreneurs in the business of delivering ambulatory services, since hospitals with their dependent employees enjoy a broad spectrum of medical decision making authority.

An important reason is the limitations of scientific knowledge of applied medicine with the necessary orientation toward the individual case. An additional reason is the obligation to practice medicine. This obligation to practice medicine clashes directly with the uncertainties of human reality, which, even with mathematical reliability, allows only limited ability to judge human behaviour. Therefore, there exists a discretionary power, which can border on arbitrary conclusions. This favours different – sometimes even contradictory – possibilities: either, too much or, too little is done.

This not only applies to indications, the rationale for the appropriateness of a particular therapy, but also to the various methods with which medical measures are implemented. Within the existing legal guidelines and framework, physicians are free to make whatever decision they choose.(4) However: a non-indicated treatment can be considered bodily harm and thereby unlawful.

The limited scientific basis of applied medicine also manifests itself in false diagnoses with sufficient frequency that it cannot be ignored. Similar to a study by the Harvard Medical School, the Medical University Clinic in Kiel came to the following conclusions based on autopsies: between 1959 and 1989 the rate of false diagnosis varied from 7 to 12 percent. Also, 25 percent of the cases proved to be lacking any diagnosis.

The most common errors in diagnosing were lung-artery embolisms, myocardial infarction, malignancy and infections.(5) In European university clinics, of cases determined to have a patho-genetic cause of death, 35 to 40 percent are at obvious discrepancy with the results of autopsies. In these cases, the clinical diagnosis were not determined to be completely false, but needing correction, needing additional information and generally needing improvement.

Despite this realization, the frequency of autopsies in Germany is decreasing. The autopsy rate on patients who died in a German hospital went from 14.6 percent in 1980 to 1.2 percent in 1995.(6)

The Institute of Medicine of the National Academy of Science in Washington, D.C. has come to more far-reaching conclusions. It reports that only 4 percent of all medical services, delivered daily, are based on scientifically proven evidence. 45 percent of health services are questionable and 51 percent have no basis in scientific proof in the strict sense.(7) Another estimation is that only 10 to 20 percent of all recommended therapies are founded on "hard" scientific data. (8)

Additionally, the Expert Council of the World Health Organization, in 1996, came to the conclusion, "that only 20 percent of all medical services are supported by empirical evidence, while in the case of the other 80 percent the evidence varies from more or less plausible to non existent." (9) The professional German language journal for internists, Medizinische Klinik, examined the results of 132 original controlled studies published between 1979 and 1996. The examined works unsatisfactorily fulfilled the criteria of a methodologically controlled study. In only 6 of 132 works, was information about the number of cases a precondition to be able to reach statistically meaningful conclusions.(10)

Differing medical decisions

This individual, uncertain, sensitive and complex area is susceptible to external influences. Money, competition, legal security, career expectations, economic existence and employment security, can easily influence the decision process for a particular treatment, either consciously or unconsciously.

Within the practice of medicine there is increasing competition for market share.(11) There are numerous examples of how varying medical decisions for the same morbidity status cannot be explained by "medical facts".

Many doctors still see the contradiction between economic pressure and the delivery of services to an individual patient as insoluble. Cost-benefit calculations that stem from a utilitarian way of thinking still find little acceptance.

At the same time, one must realize that external selection criteria enter into a physician's decisions. A study on this topic found,

"One can observe a gradual use of age limitations, as well as other criteria including insurance status, occupation, education and social status. In the words of one actor: 'This would never be said openly'. None of these criteria is legitimized morally, legally or medically" (12)

In Germany the criterion remains that which is "medically necessary". This is not only a biological factor, but is also – in a significant way – determined by the specific context of the society and normative as well as distributional premises.

What is medically necessary?

Because of the criteria for "medically necessary" in the delivery of medical services, medicine is spoken of as a science, since the "quality and effectiveness of the services have to reflect the current state of medical knowledge."(13)

This formulation in the legal code can be traced back to the earliest laws, which still apply today, stating that illness is a condition requiring treatment. Thereby the power of defining what is medically necessary is placed on the medical profession. This is closely associated with the "need to be efficient." (14)

That means:

"The services must be deemed adequate, practical and efficient. They are not permitted to go beyond what is necessary. Benefits that are not necessary or economically efficient, cannot be anticipated by the insured, are not allowed to be delivered by the provider and cannot be covered by the sickness funds".

This means, that what is medically necessary is paid by the statutory health insurance system. What is deemed not be medically necessary, must be paid by the patient.

In the background of the debate of what constitutes medical necessity is the actual health policy discussion, whether to divide the catalogue of services covered by the sickness funds into "basic" and "choice" categories. The list of "choice" services could then be offered in a competitive market with co-payments.

All serious attempts at defining which services should be considered "choice" have failed. The limitation of contract physicians' income through global budgets (1997) started a public conflict amongst the contract doctors, what was considered necessary and what was not, what would be paid by the sickness funds and what would require payment from the patient. Services, which were earlier considered necessary and required no additional payment, suddenly became unnecessary.

The discretionary power and the question of necessity form the basis of a discussion over "unnecessary operations", superfluous heart catheters and balloon dilations of the coronary arteries or avoidable hospital referrals.

Remedial measures should be rational and be able to be monitored through practice guidelines, protocols and standards until true evidence-based medicine is achieved, which has the goal of replacing – or to complementing – pragmatic medical experience with scientifically secured research results.

Trust or contractual relationship

For some time, medical institutions have been confronted with hard neoliberal economic concepts as a result of a soft scientific foundation. The expansion of the market, competition and profitability will deeply change the doctor-patient relationship. Today, the already fragile relationship based on trust (15) will more and more be altered into a mercantile contractual relationship.

The completion of a contract is, however, not exactly an expression of trust, but more one of mistrust. It is intended to secure a risky relationship between strangers, while trust has the pre-condition of a close personal relationship and familiarity on the part of both parties.

Trust makes possible the communication of intimate information that – since it can be essential for medical treatment – and it is also the basis of the need for confidentiality. Beyond this, a trusting relationship is built on an unequal basis, in which expertise, based on best knowledge, is expected to care for the welfare of the layman.

One can therefore rely on the competence of the expert, can count on his good intentions, can believe what he has to say, and trust him. Trust is a pre-condition for responsible actions. Services, which are delivered on the basis of trust, are similar to credible promises, grounded in reliability and well meaning. Trust cannot be bought.

By contrast, contracts are expressions of current law. They represent explicitly agreed upon conditions and tasks with corresponding responsibilities. In particular, the development of the market and of private property characterizes the nature of contract law. In the market, owners appear as formally equal proprietors and exchange commodities for negotiated and agreed upon prices. In fact, sellers and purchasers seek their own advantage.

In any given medical treatment, the legal relationship between patients and providers – namely, physicians and hospitals – are determined by the common law, court rulings and social law. Although the services that a physician delivers to a patient are based on his attempt to help and heal, they don't always lead to the desired healing effect. This cannot be required from a physician.

Even more, the doctor owes the patient a treatment based on recognized medical science. Although the doctor is required to explain his recommendations and respect the patients' wishes, patients often willingly follow the recommendations of their physician without fully realizing the associated risks. In such situations, the patient trusts the doctor in good faith.

With the increasing commercialisation of the doctor-patient relationship, doctors are more and more expected to offer special, measurable services at a fixed price. This increasingly takes on the characteristic of a commodity or service, produced and distributed under competitive conditions.

Correspondingly, the patient is transitioned more and more into a customer or client, one from, whom profits can be made. And the "best customer" as a rule, is the one from whom the most profit can be attained. Under such conditions, patients may be served as "royal customers", however, no longer treated as sick individuals. (16)

The more competition increases, the more the purchasing power of the patient is expected. A mercantile incentive is achieved, such that more services are delivered according to patients' wishes as opposed to patients' needs. The services are oriented more on what the patient as laymen understands as quality. The quality of medical treatment is reduced to short-term patient satisfaction. And through satisfaction, "customers" are obtained.

Patient satisfaction as the guiding principle for medical treatment

The uncertain footing of treatment oriented toward patient satisfaction becomes apparent, among others, in the case of prescription writing. In this context, physicians often refer to the expectations ("greediness") of their patients. Many patients demand medication and place the physician under pressure. When patients fail to receive a prescription, they are dissatisfied and feel they have been treated poorly.

The extent to which this expectation for medication has an influence was investigated during the beginning of the 1990s in two similar studies in Australia and England. An astonishing observation was made: more important than the expectation of the patient was the physician's opinion whether or not their patient desired medication in explaining the rate of prescription writing. General Practitioners who believed that their patient expected a prescription had a 10 times higher rate of prescription writing as those physicians who assumed their patients did not expect a prescription.(17)

Moreover, the expectation of the patient and the estimation of the physician were in no way identical. The false estimations by the doctors were considerable. 13 percent of patients whose physicians believed they expected prescriptions did not, in fact, expect a prescription.(18)

In the meantime, the phenomenon of satisfaction has developed in industrialized countries into a far-reaching "culture of satisfaction", which today – especially in the USA – represents the position of the majority and no longer the minority, writes J. K. Galbraith (19).

Throughout history, one can learn "that individuals – also groups – who are favoured with respect to their economic, social, and political situation, put in place social values and promote the continuance of political systems from which they themselves profit the most. This is done, even when overwhelming proof exists, that the opposite is correct. It is only in the belief of the favoured, that these continual, however, short term goals lead to satisfaction and thereby ensure that the economic and political trends follow. The political market is very receptive for these trends, ensuring satisfaction and security.

And there will always be social groups, which serve this market and harvest its bounty in the form of money or public accolades." (20)

The "hidden persuaders" of the market and its solicitive potential, will concentrate on exactly those patient groups whose satisfaction is sought. Profitability and commercial self-interest, the genuine concomitant phenomena of economic competition, are demonstratively pushed into the foreground.

From the patient perspective, services are viewed increasingly from the aspect of the ability to sue (malpractice) and increased control (second opinion). Increasingly, the patient expects a guarantee. Defensive medicine is expanding out of fear of liability. This means, more and more diagnostic measures are being taken, even when there are no scientific therapeutic consequences. The phrase "diagnostic overkill" is making the rounds.

Beyond this, the direction of the decision structure in the doctor-patient relationship is changing: while today, medical necessity and the severity of illness are considered the decisive factors, under the requirements of competition, economic criteria are increasingly important. Economic criteria are raised to the level of triage criteria.

Ethical aspects: Health is a Human Right

With the growing commercialisation of the delivery of medical care, well-informed patients find themselves in a difficult and unforeseeable situation. What is the meaning of medical information given during a doctor's visit, such as "that is not medically necessary", "the risks associated with this treatment is in your case too high", "and this therapy is ineffective in your situation"?

Does it mean, the treatment is not medically justified – or does it simply mean it is too expensive? How does a patient know why the doctor has given this advice? Is it indeed the best choice of therapy for this illness? Are alternative therapies being withheld? Are such recommendations dependent perhaps on the income, the career, or the job security of the physician or even the economic solvency of the hospital, which determines the stock prices and the dividends? Thanks to shareholder value. Or has the doctor just been informed that his budget has been exceeded?

This demonstrates the limits of microeconomic rationality in delivering health care that is perhaps profitable, but no longer reflects the intentions of our civilization. The pressure of economic competition places the microeconomic model in danger of ignoring its destructive potential, leading to a cultural change in medicine.(21)

The increasing commercialisation does not appear to be a problem only for the practical side of medicine, but also for medical research. Jeffrey Baker of Albright College in Pennsylvania puts forth the thesis that apparently too few scientists take the necessary precautions. Patient rights are not sufficiently protected.

After the sensational death of a genetically treated adolescent, several research projects at American institutions were discontinued or even prohibited. Baker sees the origins of this development, like many others, in the increasing commercialisation of medical research. Results must be achieved within a short time frame. Comprehensive and fair explanations to the clinical trial participants are time consuming and, in the end, could scare away subjects. On the other hand, many researchers have a financial interest in the firm that produces the product being clinically tested. They have a direct interest, to include as many subjects in the study as possible. (22)

Health researchers are witnessing an increasing dependence on economic pressure. In the U.S., it costs $500 million to bring a new drug to market. Private research and academic institutions compete for a part of the available financial resources, the majority of which goes to private institutions.

"This situation allows the industry to determine the study design, the access to raw data, as well as how the results are interpreted – in a way that is not always in the best interest of the researcher, the study subjects or scientific research methods. It has been reported that, in certain instances when study results were inconsistent with the sponsors expectations, the results were not allowed to be published." (23)

The German pharmacologist Peter Schönhöfer argues in a similar manner. He sees the quality of the German health care system threatened by the withdrawal of state support of clinical research.

"There are no longer funds available for critical, innovative research. Researchers, who are primarily oriented toward quality research in Germany no longer have an existential basis, since the sponsors are only interested in product, or marketing research. The rapid loss of critical potential is accompanied with a drastic loss of quality of clinical research." (24)

The lack of societal debate under the requirements of commercialisation, leads to increased alienation in the doctor-patient relationship and in research, and according to Jürgen Habermas, this is also true for society as a whole. He writes:

"Effects of alienation tend to appear, when areas of life that function on agreed upon social norms, value orientations, and societal communication become dominated by money and bureaucracy."

And furthermore:

"A growing societal complexity does not necessarily lead to effects of alienation. It can also open new options and possibilities for learning... Social pathologies only appear as a consequence of invasive commercial relationships and bureaucratic regulations into public and private spheres. These pathologies are not limited to personality structures, but also on the continuation of meaning and the dynamic of societal integration."(25)

At the moment, we find ourselves in a difficult, involved situation. It leads to a climate, which is influenced by two currents:

The knowledge of scientific medicine regarding stem cells and molecular biological associations as well as the corresponding therapeutic treatments is impressive. Medical technology seems to know no limits. In the meantime, it has been pushed to the level of the gene. With these media-effective events, society's understanding of illness and health is beginning to shift – admittedly with grave consequences.

On the other hand is the economic development in the health system. In almost all areas of the health care system, there is a feverish search for the possibility of applying self-regulating market mechanisms, economic competition and microeconomic constructs. In this way, economic profitability tends to suppress medical necessity, the main criterion for physicians' work.

The combination of biology and economy can lead to fatal results when human nature is reduced to "homo biologicus" and "homo economicus". No attempt will be made here to describe the specific experiences of German history, since today these relationships present themselves in a different light under different political conditions. But it is necessary to be aware of these developments and to influence health policy in a way that society is protected from the uncontrolled and self-determining combination of biology and economy.

This set of problems leads to the conclusion that a society must have sectors oriented towards the common welfare that are protected and cannot be entrusted to the blind power of the market and the deregulated strength of competition.

'Protected sectors' refers to the way vulnerable groups are dealt with, to vulnerable social goals such as solidarity and social justice, or to vulnerable communication structures (i.e. physician-patient-relationship). Indeed, they form the basis of the European social model. This quality needs to be accepted.

The quantity, the magnitude and the extent of such a welfare-oriented safety net, is dependent on the existing strengths of the representative social interest groups. The fields of illness and health are by no means peripheral or marginal societal phenomena. In fact, the right to health is a human right.

Occasionally, the shameless instrumentalisation of basic social values for disguised partial interests leads to the false assumption, that the meaning of human rights lies in their abuse.

But human rights are not to be commercialised; they don't lend themselves to being marketed, without destroying their meaning.

REFERENCES

1 Compare with: N. Schmacke, Konzentration auf die "wirklich wichtigen Leistungen"?, in: Die Ersatzkasse, H. 11, 1997, S. 398.

2 H.-U. Deppe, Zur sozialen Anatomie des Gesundheitssystems, Neoliberalismus und Gesundheitspolitik in Deutschland, Frankfurt a.m. 2000, S. 209-258.

3 T.C. James, The Patient-Physician Relationship: Convenant or Contract? In: Mayo Clin. Proc., Vol. 71, 1996, S. 917-918.

4 Sachverständigenrat für die Konzertierten Aktion im Gesundheitswesen, Bedarfsgerechtigkeit und Wirtschaftlichkeit, Gutachten 2000/2001, Bd. III, ausführliche Zusammenfassung, S. 29.

5 Ch. Schafii, W. Kirch, Thema: Fehldiagnosen, in: Der Kassenarzt, Heft 40, 1993, S. 34f. It needs to be considered, that university clinics treat patients with the most severe and complicated illnesses. Also, autopies are done when diagnoses are unclear.

6 E B, Obduktionen – Bedenklicher Rückgang, in: Deutsches Ärzteblatt, H. 13, 2000, S. 685.

7 Nach: M.J.Field, K.N. Lohr (Hrsg.), Guidelines For Clinical Practice: From Development to Use, Washington 1992.

8 R. Volkert, Der lange Weg in die Praxis, in: Deutsches Ärzteblatt, H. 27, 1998, S. 1368.

9 Die Ortskrankenkasse, H. 17-18, 1997, S. 563.

10 Deutsches Ärzteblatt, H. 13, 1999, S. 639.

11 R. Flöhl, Die Chirurgie kämpft um Marktanteile, in: Frankfurter Allgemeine Zeitung vom 14. April 1999.

12 E. Kuhlmann, „Zwischen zwei Mahlsteinen" – Ergebnisse einer empirischen Studie zur Verteilung knapper medizinischer Ressourcen in ausgewählten klinischen Settings, in: G. Feuerstein, E. Kuhlmann (Hrsg.), Rationierung im Gesundheitswesen, Wiesbaden 1998, S. 72.

13 §2 SGB V.

14 §12 SGB V.

15 St. Busse, Chr. Schierwagen, Vertrauen, in: J. Sandkühler (Hrsg.), Europäische Enzyklopädie zu Philosophie und Wissenschaften, Hamburg 1990, Bd. 4, S. 719ff.

16 Compare with: J. Wertheimer, Die Universität bedient keine Kunden, sondern erzieht Menschen, in: Frankfurter Rundschau , Decembre 4, 1997.

17 J. Cockburn, S. Pit, Prescribing Behaviour in Clinical Practice: Patients´Expections and Doctors´Perception of Patients´Expections – a Questionary Study, in: BMJ, Vol. 315, 1997, S. 521.

18 N. Britten, O. Ukoumune, The Influence of Patients´Hopes of Receiving a Prescription on Doctors´Perception and the Decision to Prescribe: a Questionnaire Survey, in: BMJ, Vol. 315, 1997, S. 1509. Zu ähnlichen Ergebnissen für Deutschland kommt: E. Lippert-Urbanke, Primärärztliche Arzneimittelverordnung: Wechselseitige Erwartungen von Arzt und Patient, Diss.med. Universität Göttingen 1997.

19 J.K. Galbraith, Die Herrschaft der Bankrotteure, Hamburg 1992, S. 21ff.

16 *Commercialisation or solidarity?*

Ibid., S.12.
H.-U. Deppe, Vor einer Kulturwende in der Medizin, in: Soziale Sicherheit, H. 5, 1999, S. 183-185.
St. Sahm, Patienten nur unzureichend geschützt, in: Frankfurter Allgemeine Zeitung vom 15. November 2000.
St. Mertens, Viel heisse Luft, in: Deutsches Ärzteblatt, H. 46, 2001, S. 2573.
P. Schönhöfer, Missbrauch, Betrug und Verschwendung, in: H.-U. Deppe, W. Burkhardt (Hrsg.), Solidarische Gesundheitspolitik, Hamburg 2002, S. 119.

Social care policies, national government and private interests
JANE LETHBRIDGE

This paper will examine some of the characteristics of social care policies in the context of different national systems and how private sector
interests are responding to policy changes.

Many national policy changes in financing and delivery of social care
services have been triggered by the perceived view that the increasing
size of the older population will cause an expansion in demand for social
care services for older people. Although services are still funded by taxation in many countries, some countries have introduced new systems of
long term care insurance and co-payments.

There has been a transfer of services from the public sector to the
private and voluntary sectors but municipal and local state authorities
remain responsible for commissioning and purchasing social care services in many countries. There has also been a decline in the number of
care homes with a corresponding rise in home care services, with the
private sector, becoming the dominant provider in many countries.

A new type of funding provision involves the government giving
money directly to service users so that they can purchase services to
meet their own care needs individually. The impact of these arrangements on users of services, the care workforce and private companies is
only just beginning to be understood.

The paper will also assess the relatively new social care model being
introduced in countries of Central and Eastern Europe and to what
extent private companies are becoming involved in provision.

The paper will conclude with a discussion of the future regulatory role of government.

What is social care?

Social care work can be defined as "activities that provide assistance or supervision for someone requiring support in daily life, which can be delivered at home, in the community or in a variety of settings". Those being cared for include children, adults with long term chronic conditions, people with physical or learning disabilities, people with mental health problems and older people. This paper will examine care workers involved in a social model of care for children and for older people.

Childcare and the care of older people have traditionally been studied as two separate issues although this is beginning to change. One of the reasons for this separation in research is the different administrative and cultural understanding of the extent of public responsibility for care (Rosgaard, 2002).

In Nordic countries, social care covers public care provided for everyone who needs it — older people, children, and people with disabilities. In the United Kingdom, social care is limited to care for older people, people with disabilities and adults with mental health problems.

This paper will initially address childcare and the care of older people separately but, will also draw some comparisons between these two forms of social care, particularly in the ways in which state, family, private and voluntary sectors operate.

The role of the welfare state also shapes care as an activity and a set of social relations (Daly and Lewis, 2000). Many typologies have been developed to examine different welfare systems, which may be defined, for example, in relation to the expected role of the family in caring for older people and children, or tax based and social insurance funding (Esping-Andersen, 1990; Alber, 1995).

Jenson identified three types of welfare state programmes that all influence the way in which care is defined and delivered:

● Programmes that "redistribute the risk of differential needs for care", for example family policy for bringing up children;

● Programmes that aim to improve the quality of care by regulating providers or professionalizing care;

● Programmes that provide pensions and allowances to reduce dependency (Jenson, 2002, p. 70).

Government involvement in social care occurs in several forms: funding for care services, which are delivered directly to a person in their own home or in a residential home; payments to informal carers, known as a "carer's allowance"; funding directly to people needing care, who can then purchase services from local social care agencies.

The government role in the direct provision of social care is declining in many countries and the provision of social care services, even when funded by the public sector, is increasingly provided by the private and non-profit sector.

There are several types of social care for older people in Europe: care provided at home; in residential homes; and care provided in specific types of sheltered housing. Home care consists of different types of support, for example, cleaning, bathing, dressing of wounds, and shopping, that enable an older person to continue to live in their own home.

Social care provided in residential homes is for older people who can no longer live alone and need some combination of nursing and social care. Increasingly new residential schemes are being built by private, and in some cases public-private partnerships that provide accommodation for older people and access to centralized care support when needed.

Social care workers may work in residential homes or provide care to older people at home or in sheltered housing schemes. They may be employed directly by the public sector, usually a local authority or municipality, but increasingly they are employed, either directly or self-employed, by the private or non-profit sectors.

Childcare services are delivered through daycare centres, childcare centres, nursery schools, pre- and after-school centres and family households. In countries where there is a greater public sector or non-governmental provision, workers are directly employed in childcare centres, nursery schools and pre- and after-school centres.

In countries, often where childcare is provided predominantly by the private sector, for example, the United States or the United Kingdom, many childcare workers are employed by the private sector. Childminders, babysitters and nannies are three major categories of child care workers that are employed directly by a household or family, or are self-employed. They take care of children either in their own homes or those of the children. Babysitters are paid on an hourly basis and do a range of activities. Nannies are often full time, sometimes live with the family and provide a range of services from childcare to housework.

Childcare and pre-school care is increasingly being characterized as having both caring and educational components, which is also influencing whether childcare policy is considered as part of educational or welfare policy. During the last decade there have been examples of governments moving responsibility from welfare/health departments to education departments, for example in England and Sweden. These departmental changes have implications for how the services are organized and delivered, and the way in which care workers are trained and paid (Cohen et al., 2004).

The demand for paid care workers to care for older people and children is strongly influenced by demographic factors and increased women's participation in the paid labour force. For older people, increased women's participation in the paid labour force affects the number of unpaid carers, often women, who are able to care for older relatives. The provision of parental leave has a strong influence on the demand for childcare facilities. This can range from very limited parental leave to three years paid leave in Hungary (Korintus and Moss, 2004). The demand for childcare is also influenced by employment policies, which seek to encourage increased female participation in the workforce.

Daly and Lewis (2000) present a concept of contemporary social care that looks at social care infrastructure, the political economy of provision between the family, market, state and voluntary/community sectors and the contribution of each sector to the organization of care. This will help to understand the institutional characteristics that determine the organization of care across sectors, and the politics that accompany these differences. This paper will go on to explore:

● How national governments have influences social care in the last decade

● How private interests have become more involved in social care

● The impact of these changes on services users and care workers

The material for this paper has been drawn from research reports on care and care workers. Academic databases have been used to identify published research. There have been several large research programmes in Europe that have been examining both social care for older people and childcare.

The results of these research programmes provide important new material that help to understand how care work is changing. They also show that much more research is needed to understand and shape future care work.

Industry wide analyses, company annual reports and other company materials have been used to understand multinational company strategies. Reports from international and national agencies, policy documents and trade union surveys of working conditions have also been used to provide a global view of care policies.

Other sources that have been consulted include national newspapers, trade union reports, and non-governmental research.

Forms of financing and payment for social care for older people

In the past two decades, policies for the provision of care for older people have moved from advocating solely family care to a combination of small scale institutional settings and community care, with a mix of public and private responsibility. Home care has expanded as part of community care. National policies that promote market mechanisms in social care have been introduced since the early 1980s in Europe as well as North America and Australia, which has led to the setting up of internal markets, the introduction of user fees, the privatization of some care services and an overall shift from public to private provision (Go, 1998).

In the UK the Community Care Act (1992) promoted subcontracting from local authorities to private providers by separating local authority purchasing and providing functions. The Community Care Direct Payment Act also led to increased home care provision. The UK also introduced "attendance allowances" as payment for carers who previously would have provided unpaid, informal care. The introduction of care allowance programmes was determined more by the aim of allowing older people to remain independent rather than before the goals of valuing informal caring (Jenson, 2002).

The 1992 Adel reforms in Sweden have led to an expansion of private sector provision with the contracting out of long-term care facilities, home-care services, meal and transport services.

In Germany, a Long-term Care Insurance Law was introduced in 1994, which introduced universal insurance to cover the costs of long-term care. In this case the provision of long term insurance has led to the expansion of private sector provision as a result of private companies having been given subsidies to build new facilities, while subsidies for non-governmental organizations were reduced. In Japan, similar policy changes have led to an expansion of private social care provision (Go, 1998).

Changes in the healthcare sector have also led to national social care policy changes due to the mutual dependence of these sectors. The attempts to limit the number of older people in acute hospital beds in some countries, for example the United Kingdom and Sweden, has created a new category of 'intermediate' care.

Since 2003, local authorities in England are penalized if they are unable to provide appropriate care and accommodation through the Community Care (Delayed Discharge) Act (Pollock, 2004). This has led to local authorities changing both the organization of social care and the way it is priced. Social care is now more dependent on service provision from profit and non-profit providers, creating new opportunities to charge for care services.

Many of these policy changes have emphasized consumer choice and the concept of the service user as a "purchaser". Although many of these changes are presented government as part of a process of empowering service users, there has been an element of cost cutting. In some countries there has been an underlying assumption that individually managed care would be cheaper than institutional residential care.

The impact of these new systems of funding and financing of social care vary in different European countries according to the welfare state system already in place, and the measures taken to reform it.

There has been an expansion of home care in many countries where systems of social care funding have changed. With an increase in individually assessed care packages, there is a rising demand for care services delivered at home. At the same time there has also been an increase in medical care services that can be delivered at home, for example, cancer treatments and renal dialysis. Trained nurses and other specialized health workers deliver these services.

Although they are not going to be considered in this paper, it is important to be aware of this parallel development of medical home care services for the private sector because it will affect the future of home-care services.

Older people and people with disabilities, in some countries, are being given money from public funding to purchase the services that they need. In some cases, user organisations consider that this gives people with disabilities the opportunity to organise the services to meet their own specific needs. However, where, older people do not feel able to purchase their own services, social workers do on their behalf, as a protective practice.

To enable people to purchase their own social care services, the services had to be costed and priced, which started the process of commodifying social care services. This is illustrated by the case of Denmark, where the delivery of services has been influenced by changes in national policies for older people. Nursing home residents were given the right to choose which services they take up, so nursing homes were obliged to define the services that they provided and their cost (Lewinter, 2004).

The introduction of market principles to the public social care sector has resulted in many home care services becoming "business units", and having to compete with the private sector (Trydefard, 2003). Care services in municipalities have also been redefined as "care products". Methods for "measuring and securing the quality of care" have been introduced which have been drawn from the private sector and the manufacturing sector (Trydefard, 2003).

Services are provided by one of three main types of care provider: individual care workers; non-profit care services; and commercial care services. In countries where only the basic costs of care are provided by government, any extra costs have to be covered by the individual, leading to the introduction of user fees.

Forms of financing and payment for childcare

There is a growing recognition that government has a role to play in providing or subsidizing childcare, unlike social care for older people. The increasing participation of women in the labour market has increased over the last decades, with government employment policies supporting this trend. In addition, research into the value of effective child care support during the first three years of a child's life is showing that enhancing the social well-being of young children will positively influence their adult life.

Government involvement in childcare can take three forms:

● first, direct funding of childcare through government centres or subsidies to other arrangements/providers;

● secondly, government subsidies to families to offset cost of childcare, such as through tax credits or tax relief;

● and thirdly, regulation of centre based care and family care homes.

As with social care for older people, national systems of provision are influenced by historical patterns of care and ways of delivering them, for example, the use of targeted or universal provision.

In Sweden, 78% of women participate in the paid labour force with 29% of children aged 0-3 years in day care. 8.5% of families with children are at poverty level. The level of poverty of single mothers increased in the 1990s. Women are over represented in the public sector, which has more flexible and part time working arrangements, but women's employment has also been more affected by the privatization of public services (Cohen et al., 2004).

Early childhood education and care services in Sweden were largely protected by central government during the 1990s, and as such have been less affected by privatization and liberalization. Parental leave arrangements are generous (Allen, 2003).

Since 1999, 98% of municipalities are able to provide care for all children of 1 year and older within 3 months of a request. Parents also make some contribution to costs. Low income parents pay 3-4% of their childcare costs although this varies according to municipality and whether fixed or sliding fees are used (Allen, 2003).

Policy drivers

The origins of some of the changes in the way that social care is funded and delivered can be seen in policy developments at supra-regional and international levels. Childcare policies need to be seen in terms of employment policies and strategies to either increase women's participation in the paid labour force or decrease unemployment among single parents.

Policies for older people are strongly influenced by a negative view of older people which presents older people as a "burden" and unable to contribute to society. This is characterized by viewing older people as a "time bomb" that will place great pressure on existing social welfare programmes.

With a relatively smaller working population, the funds generated from taxation and other contributions to the funding of social welfare programmes will decrease.

In Europe, the Maastricht Treaty (1993) was one of the most important factors that led to the liberalization of the social care sector. One of the Maastricht Treaty criteria stated that "Member states shall avoid excessive government deficits (Article 104c.1)". Absence of a deficit was one of four criteria for entry into the Economic Monetary Union. Contracting out of services, including social care services to private or non-profit providers, was one way in which governments could reduce their deficits (PSPRU, 1997).

The influence of the European Union (EU) has also been important because of the absence of specific EU level policy on both older people and children. The overall role of the European Union in social care policy has been limited and is similar to the situation in healthcare, where the principle of subsidiarity allows national governments to develop their own social care policies. There have been some attempts by the EU to influence social care policy for both children and older people, but these have taken the form of recommendations or advice rather than binding legislation. These include Recommendations on ChildCare (92/241/EEC) adopted by the Council on 31 March 1992, which points out that lack of childcare limits women's participation in the paid labour force, but which does not provide further obligations for Member states to meet any minimum requirements (Rostgaard, 2002).

The "Green Book on European Social Policy" (1993) encouraged Member states to share responsibility for social policy implementation with voluntary organizations, social partners and local authorities.

As part of the EU Employment strategy, each Member state has to develop its own employment strategy to incorporate many groups that are not currently part of the paid labour force (EU, 1997). The provision of childcare has been recognized as an important factor in getting women back into the paid labour force. Single mothers with children have been a target group in many countries, for example, under the New Deal Programme in the United Kingdom.

The European Union is expected to have more influence on the social care sector through its internal market legislation. A new draft Services Directive (June 2004) "Services in the internal market COM(2004)" recommended that "personal social services" should be considered a Service of General Economic Interest (SGI) and as such be subject to competition law rather than a Service of General Interest (SGI) which would not be subject to competition.

One of the most important implications of this classification is that a service provider operating within the EU will be subject to the laws of its country of origin and not to those of the host country where the service is actually provided. Companies are expected to establish themselves in countries which have weak labour legislation and then expand into other European countries. This is expected to affect both the working conditions of social care workers and the quality of services provided (EPHA, 2004).

Following extensive campaigning and lobbying from a wide range of organisations, institutions and governments the Directive was abandoned in its present form. In February 2005, the Commission President Barroso announced that "As the Directive was written, it would not have been successful...This is the reason why the Commission has unanimously accepted to make changes" (CELSIG Agence Europe).

A number of developments mean that the issue of whether social care services should be classified as a Service of General Interest has not been resolved. The Altmark judgement by the European Court of Justice (ECJ) has resulted in the decision "to exclude Government support for services, such as public transport, from the term "state aid" and therefore from the tendering requirement". This is also significant for social care services. Local authorities that are currently providers of social care services will not be expected to tender these services.

There are continuing discussions on the possibility of a Framework Directive for Services of General Interest. Some of the issues emerging in these discussions can be seen in the outcomes of a conference held in June 2004 "Social Services of General Interest in the European Union – Assessing their Specificities, Potential and Needs" which outlined a number of issues that need to be considered in the context of social services as Services of General Interest (SGI).

This conference brought together the German Federal Ministry for Family Affairs, Senior Citizens, Women and Youth, the Platform of European Social NGOs and the Observatory for the Development of Social Services in Europe with the support of the European Commission. It can be seen to reflect many of the concerns felt by a range of stakeholders involved in the future development of social services.

The conference felt that the "modernisation" policies introduced to social services have been based on the assumed need to cut costs. Future modernisation of social services needs to take a wider view of how to meet the needs of people for social care services, rather than view change only in relation to budgetary reductions.

The definition and measurement of quality of services remains a difficult issue to address. Specific questions, about which stakeholders should do this, how, and at what level, need further discussion. The language of Services of General Economic Interest (SGEI) and economic performance indicators is not appropriate for social services. Social services may need a legal recognition to give them a clearer identity, which would include "appropriate modulated application of market and competition rules, according to user needs and quality of services". There are unresolved tensions between local, regional, national and EU levels of society in relation to social services. Continued participation of stakeholders, to inform the development of the EC "Communication on social and health services in the European Union", is still needed.

Changes in welfare state programmes affecting social care provision such as the introduction of payments for individuals to pay for caring services or for informal carers to be paid an allowance or wage, have contributed to the commercialization of social care delivery. Although presented as part of a process of the welfare state recognizing the rights of both carer and person needing care, these new arrangements also contribute to a system of quantifiable care services where care has become a commodity.

The European Union is contributing to this process of commercialization by making social care services subject to internal market legislation. At both supra-regional and international level, policy papers on older people consistently present older people as an economic burden. Together with policies to reduce public sector spending and promote the role of the private sector in care, the move towards commodification of care will continue. For childcare, the implications of the commodification of care services also affect the way in which childcare services are developed and delivered in systems where the private and non-profit sectors dominate.

During the last two decades, there has been an expansion in private and non-governmental provision of social care services in many European countries. This is illustrated by the decrease in numbers of residential beds provided by the public sector, often as part of municipal services. It can also be seen through the increase in the number of private sector providers of home-care services. Whilst there are clearly identifiable moves from public to private and non-governmental provision, the patterns of ownership in the private sector are diffuse.

In several European countries, large parts of national markets are dominated by a group of national companies whose ownership changes regularly. The rest of the private sector consists of many small and medium scale businesses providing residential and or home care. In most national social care markets, continual processes of merger and acquisition have been taking place in the last decade. The United Kingdom, France and the Nordic region will be discussed below.

United Kingdom

In the United Kingdom, there has been a widespread transfer of care from the public sector to the private and non-profit sector. The number of local authority residential care beds fell from 54,610 beds in 1998 to 37,210 in 2002 (Pollock, 2004). This has resulted in the expansion of the private residential and home care sector (Pollock and Price, 2001). Local authorities now purchase more home care services from the private and non-profit sector than they deliver themselves (Laing and Buisson, 2003). There has also been an increase in the demand for home care following the National Health Service and Community Care Act (1990) (Community Care Direct Payment Act), which enables older people to purchase their care directly from service providers.

The social care market in the UK is dominated by a group of five companies. Private equity, venture capitalists and business groups involved in the service sector are the main shareholders. These groups are interested in a good rate of return on their investments and change their shareholdings in these companies regularly. Apart from BUPA, these companies were set up in the 1980s and 1990s, following changes in community care legislation, and have had several changes of ownership. In 2004, three of these companies had significant changes in their shareholders.

These companies provide care services for older people, homecare services, people with disabilities and in some cases childcare. Pollock (2004) discusses the increasing size of nursing care homes. The larger the care home, the more profitable it will be because the larger companies have access to higher revenues and can generate economies of scale (Holden, 2002). Residents may feel that the larger size of homes may contribute to a sense of institutionalization and decrease in the quality of care (Pollock, 2004). Many of these companies are also becoming involved in home care.

As in the UK social care market, there have been several changes of ownership in the last 2-3 years. Private equity and venture capital also play an important role as shareholders in the social care sector. ORPEA bought a 29% share in MEDIDEP in 2003. This was sold in 2005 after pressure was placed on the Chief Executive of ORPEA to resign from the Medidep supervisory board. Several hedge or investment funds (Amber Funds Ltd, Centaurus Capital LP and Mellon HBY Alternative Strategies) had demanded his resignation. ORPEA sold its 29% share, which was bought by the investment funds, at □25.50 per share. They sold these shares shortly afterwards to Suren, another French care company, at □39.32 per share. This illustrates the short term profits to be made in the care sector, by investment companies.

Bridgepoint, a European private equity group, bought 70% of Medica France from Caisse de Depots, a Quebec fund manager for public and private pension funds. In 2003, Generale de Sante, a private healthcare company, sold 51% of its shares in its care homes to DOMUS Vi which allowed the founder, Yves Journel, to regain control (Medidep, 2003).

Most follow-up care and rehabilitation beds are still attached to public sector hospitals in France. Non-profit providers dominate the home care market in France. However, since 2001, the large private companies delivering residential care have also set up subsidiaries that deliver home care by obtaining home hospitalization licences, for example, MEDIDEP and Medica France (Medidep, 2003). In the home care market, private companies dominate the market for sale and rental of hospital equipment in the home.

Nordic region

In Sweden, there has also been a decline in the total number of nursing home beds since 1992. In 1992, there were approximately 32,000 beds, but following the ADEL reform these beds were transferred to the social care sector and to the municipalities (Trydefard, Thorslund,, 2001). There has been some transfer of beds from the public sector to the private and non-profit sectors. A Finnish trade union (KTV) survey in Sweden found that privatization has been introduced through competitive tendering, by turning public operations into joint-stock companies

Table 1: Five largest social care companies in the UK

Company	Shareholders	Beds	Turnover
Southern Cross Healthcare Ltd	(2004) Blackstone Group (2005) Blackstone Group bought Ashbourne Homes, owned by Cannon Capital Ventures	28,000	Recent expansion
BUPA Care services	Non-profit	17,631	£357m
Four Seasons Healthcare group	(2004)Alchemy venture capital group sold to Allianz Capital Partners (part of Allianz insurance group)	15,315	£105m
Craegmoor Group Ltd	(2001) Legal and General Ventures - subsequently syndicated a proportion of their interest to a number of other private equity investors including LDC (formerly Lloyds TSB Development Capital), CDP Capital, RBS Mezzanine and funds managed by JO Hambro	5,828	£125m
Westminster Healthcare Group	A public limited company until 1999 but since owned by financial institutions. Sold in 2004 by 3i to Barchester Healthcare Group	5,747	£142m

Source: Laing and Buisson, Community Care Market News November 2003
www.westminsterhealthcare.co.uk; www.craegmoor.co.uk; www.fourseasonshealthcare.co.uk www.southerncrosshealthcare.co.uk; www.blackstone.com

Table 2: Five largest social care companies in France

Company	Shareholders	Beds	Turnover
ORPEA	Dr. Marian 33% Other founders 25% Investors 10%	6541	€192 million
Medica France	Bridgepoint 70% Executives 30%	6332	€210 million
MEDIDEP	Various financial interests	4918	€250 million
Domus Vi	Yves Journel 68% Barclay Capital 24%	4499	€150 million

Source: Medidep Annual Report 2003

owned by local authorities, and by use of the "service voucher" model. This has also led to some contracting out of home care services to the private sector (Savolainen, 2004).

In Sweden in 1999, private providers delivered 9% of public care for older people, although services are still publicly funded, with users paying fees, which are means-tested (Trydefard,Thorslund, 2001). The market for social care until 12 months ago was dominated by four large companies, which are active in Norway, Sweden and Finland.

These four companies hold 50% of the social care contracts in Nordic countries. Privately operated care is more common in urban centres than in rural areas, suggesting that delivering care to geographically scattered communities is not profitable. The municipalities that have privatised services were more likely to be run by councillors from conservative political parties (Trydefard, 2003).

In Denmark, new national legislation, which was designed to eliminate the black market in domestic services, allocates subsidies for home service or housekeeping activities (Lewinter, 2004). Private firms, with as few as two people, can register to receive these subsidies. Anyone can hire a home service firm to do cleaning or shopping. The person receiving a service pays an hourly rate and the government also pays the service provider. In this way, the government is effectively subsidizing the expansion of private sector involvement in the home care sector.

Private provision of social care services has expanded in many European countries and the expansion of private provision is characterized by a group of, usually national, companies that dominate the market, accompanied by many small and medium sized enterprises. The extent of international provision is limited at the moment although there are signs that financial investors perceive the social care market as a suitable place for short-term investments.

Provision of services for childcare

The sectors providing childcare vary from country and are influenced by the arrangements for financing and supporting childcare. In Nordic countries, there is a large public sector provision. Parents pay some contribution to fees but this is dependent on income. In Spain there is an extensive private for profit provision where parents pay fees directly.

Thirty one per cent of children aged under 3 in Sweden were cared for in full or part time non-relative care in regulated family day care homes and 26.6% were cared for in public day centres. Private day care has only started to expand since 1990 and is still relatively small. Both family care homes and day care homes are subsidized and regulated. Responsibility has been moved down to municipal levels. The rationale given was to respond more to regional needs although cost cutting was also involved. As a result some municipal contracts were privatized (Cohen et al., 2004).

In the United Kingdom, there is a large private childcare sector, which has been encouraged by government childcare policies. Between 1997 and 2002, the number of children in childcare services increased by 547,000. Most of this increase in provision was through the expansion of

Name	Shareholders
Attendo	Bridgepoint Capital bought Attendo 2005
Capio Elderly Care	Capio Elderly Care sold to Attendo 2004
Carema	Orkla, Ovriga, Jarla Investeringar AB, and the Saven family
ISS Care partner	ISS sold 51% shares in 2002
	February 2005, ISS and EQT III fund (EQT) have agreed to form a joint venture taking over ISS Health Care and ISS CarePartner AB
	ISS became a private company in April 2005

private sector provision, sometimes supported by new business start-ups in disadvantaged areas (Cohen et al., 2004). The Education Act (2002) also allows schools to set up childcare and out of school activities.

Services for children under school age have been another area of expansion. By 2003, 99% of three year olds were receiving early years education, with 88% in publicly funded places (ONS, 2003). Although 88% were in publicly funded places, 57% of three year olds were in places provided by private and non-profit providers. There has also been an expansion of nursery place by private providers.

At the moment there are identifiable national markets for social care and childcare which each tend to be dominated by 4-5 large national companies although they are also characterized by large numbers of small operators. Companies are increasingly involved in several dimensions of care: residential care for highly dependent older people, care for adults with psychiatric/neurological conditions, home care, and residential accommodation sometimes with access to care facilities.

In the United Kingdom, care companies are also becoming involved in childcare. These are significant trends when examining the presence of multinational companies in the care sector. Cohen et al (2004) argue that nurseries and homes for older people (in the United Kingdom) have "come to exemplify the liberal welfare regime's emphasis on private provision and market solutions, in which services are treated like any other private product for which there is a demand" (Cohen et al., 2004:72).

Multinational companies

The changing nature of social care provision and the increasing trend towards both privatization and commodification has presented some multinational companies with new opportunities. Demographic trends suggest a growing demand for care services for older people and companies have identified potential new markets. However, this has not yet resulted in a major expansion by multinational companies into social care. Both childcare and social care work are labour intensive, and as many companies have found in the last decade, do not always generate profits. This section will identify some of movements of multinational companies into social care, childcare and broader investments for services for older people.

Childcare provision

In many European countries, the public sector is still the main provider of childcare services. The expansion of government support for childcare in the United Kingdom has provided opportunities for several types of private company to move into the childcare market. Private equity and venture capital trusts are involved in investing in private childcare companies. Companies already providing social care for older people are buying childcare companies, for example, the Four Seasons Group in the United Kingdom. There have also been recent movements of US childcare companies into the UK market, for example, the UK arm of the US company Kindercare was acquired by Kidsunlimited, a UK childcare company.

BUPA is a UK based non-profit company that was set up in 1947 in the United Kingdom (UK), to provide health insurance and healthcare services for privately insured patients. In the last 15 years, it has expanded into Europe and Asia to provide primary and acute care, often because the company was unable to expand into acute care within the UK, circumscribed by the NHS. However since 1990, in the UK, it has expanded extensively into residential care homes and nursery services where public sector provision is limited or has been reduced. Care services for older people and children contribute most to the company's profits (BUPA, 2003)

Broader investments

There are signs that both national and multinational companies are beginning to explore the feasibility of providing a range of services connected with ageing and social care. As mentioned in relation to national markets, the clearest model is the "assisted living concept" which draws a range of services, including social care, security systems, into a residential complex. Social care will be provided but may not be the dominant activity. This is a model, which has been developed in North America, but which is also being tested in the Nordic region and the United Kingdom.

In the Nordic region, the concept of "assisted care" for a company focuses as much on the investment in property than on the direct provision of social care. They are usually set up by an alliance of property developers, investors, social care providers and sometimes a municipal authority. Each housing unit has a kitchen and bathroom but also shares some common facilities.

They are often serviced by municipal home care services, which may be contracted out to private providers. These schemes are often built with public subsidy and residents have a tenancy agreement with rent calculated on a sliding scale. People have to be assessed by the municipality. Since the introduction of this legislation in 1997 in Denmark, there has been a decline in the number of nursing homes and an increase in assisted living schemes (Lewinter, 2004).

This trend may also be supported by changes in the way in which social care services for older people are paid for, moving towards a clearer breakdown of what services cost and older people being able to pay for specific services directly. This approach can be illustrated by the activities that Attendo Care, a Swedish multinational company, provides in three divisions.

One division provides products and systems that "improve the efficiency of providing care to older people and people with disabilities", for example, care phones or response systems. A second division helps to develop monitoring centres that become the focus of the organization of care and support. A third division provides more conventional forms of social care: nursing homes; sheltered housing; homecare. This division also provides what it describes as "over the counter" care packages to local authorities or individuals (Attendo, 2003 www.attendo.se). At the moment, the social care division is the most profitable division, which may be explained by the size of its acquisitions in the last four years.

Player and Pollock (2001) also identify the growing links between property investments and care homes in the UK. In 2004, the UK Treasury published a consultation paper on the development real estate investment trusts (REITs), which are a well established form of property investment in North America (www.hm-treasury.gov.uk).

The liberalization of social care, as seen through the introduction of an internal market within the public sector for public social care services, the contracting out and privatization of many social care services, has led to the expansion of the private social care sector in many countries. However, multinational companies have not yet expanded significantly into these national social care markets. What expansion there has been, has been slow and often short term.

The interest that private equity and venture capital investors have in both social care and childcare suggest that investments can be made in the short term with some expectations that both markets are likely to expand in the future. The increase in private companies involved in property for older people suggests that companies consider that property investments are more likely to generate profits than care service provision. In the long-term, this can be considered as an argument for public sector provision of care services.

Care workers in the workforce

The proportion of care workers as a percentage of the total workforce varies from country to country. Nordic countries have relatively high levels with Denmark (10%), Sweden (9%) and the Netherlands (7%). In the UK, care workers form 5% of the workforce with lower levels in Spain and Hungary (3%). The majority of care workers in any country are women, often 90% (Cameron, 2003). In the UK, women make up 90% of the care workforce, which is based mostly in the independent/private sector.

Labour market security

There is an increasing demand for all types of care workers. A growing number of workers are recruited from abroad because of a shortage of workers willing to work within the care sector. Only in Denmark where there is a "core" pedagogy worker, is there a growing interest in this care occupation (Cameron et al 2003).

Gender plays an important role in defining care with the majority of care workers being women. Men are also being encouraged to enter care work for both children and older people, although the percentage of male care workers is still small in all countries. Denmark has the highest proportion (14%) of male childcare workers, but the majority of men work in out-of-schools services rather than services for children from 0-3 years (Cameron et al., 2003).

Migrant labour, which is often insecure in terms of visa or residency status, is a growing segment of the care labour force. Migrant women are increasingly providing care services in childcare and care of older people as part of a global transfer of female labour from low to higher income countries. Debates about welfare state gender issues and the crisis of care have not addressed the role of migrant women in the provision of care services (Kofman, 2004; Yeates, 2004).

In many countries, the majority of social care workers are aged over 40. For example, most professional workers in the home care sector in many European countrie are between 40 and 60 years old and will soon be retiring and leaving the paid labour force. This has implications for the provision of social care in the long term.

Where care allowances are paid directly to the care-giver, these new systems of social care payments have led to a transfer of care from the informal to the formal sectors. Previously, informal care-givers have become part of the paid labour force, which has also changed family relationships (Jenson, 2002). However there is no impact on the local labour market because these care workers are family members who would be providing care whether or not they were paid.

Pay, terms and conditions

Both the social care and childcare sector are characterized by low pay in many countries, with variations between countries. Care workers in Denmark and Sweden have higher pay and status than in other countries in Europe. However, a trade union survey found that in Sweden, wages for women in caring, nursing, cleaning and food preparation have either remained unchanged or declined. Pensions, holiday pay and other benefits have also declined or become more restricted following privatization (Savolainen, 2004).

In other countries, where allowances are paid directly to informal carers, middle-aged women are able to enter the paid labour force by joining a social security scheme. However the extent of their incorporation into the paid labour force is often limited to being part of a small sub-section of the labour market characterized by insecurity and low pay (Ungerson, 2003).

Employers of childcare workers such as babysitters and nannies do not always pay statutory contributions. Workers in residential care homes for older people and home care workers, where there is a high turnover of workers, are also subject to limited income security because they have temporary or part time jobs, and have limited entitlements to other benefits. Migrant workers working in social care are not always integrated into the social security system. The lack of formal integration into the social security system will affect the long-term income of these workers. Even if part time or temporary workers are paid the same hourly rates as permanent staff, they are often not eligible for the same holidays, sick pay or pensions. This also has important implications for the long-term income of the women workers (Centre for Public Services, 1997).

Contracts

Contracts within the sector are often short term and part time for social care and childcare workers. Those working within the public sector are likely to have contracts ensuring more stability. For example, both social care and childcare workers in Denmark or Sweden have higher levels of employment security.

The availability of cash for care work also can stimulate the expansion of non-regulated, unskilled, untrained and undocumented labour. This new type of care worker is often not covered by social rights and employment regulations. Ungerson (2003), writing about the impact of carers' allowances on families in Italy found, that of those who employed a care worker, all had employed workers without rights of residence who lived locally. Of the care workers interviewed, only one care worker had residence rights in Italy.

In Austria, where care allowances are also paid directly to people needing care, a major voluntary organization, Caritas, has become involved as an employer of the care worker/giver who may be a relative. In this way, the relative can access social security rights, holiday pay, and a contract of employment. In many cases it also raises the self-esteem of the care worker who had often moved from informal caring within the family to being paid for care work.

The payment of care subsidies to care workers has facilitated the employment of undocumented foreign care workers in Austria to such an extent that agencies have been set up to organize it (Ungerson, 2003). Migrant workers are recruited, from Hungary and Skovakia, as temporary labour in Austria, by recruitment agencies. Older people often employ two care workers, one to provide 24-hour care for 2 weeks and the second to provide similar 24-hour care for the following two weeks. The migrant care workers live with the older person that they are caring for when in Austria. This enables care workers to maintain work in one country as well as returning to their home countries regularly.

In the UK, there is a trend towards casual work in the care sector to ensure 24 hour, 7 day a week cover, especially among large providers. "Care assistants rank as one of the lowest paid jobs in the UK...Living-in is a solution to the 24 hour-demands of care work, and live-in care workers are particularly prone to working excessive hours"

This makes care workers vulnerable to owners of care homes, dependent on them for accommodation, telephone and other facilities (Anderson, Rogaly, 2005). In Canada, homecare workers in the public sector have better terms and conditions than home care workers in the private sector where tenure is shorter and wages lower.

Workers in the private sector are less likely to receive pay for meetings related to management or administration. They are also more likely to feel underemployed because of the way the work is organised and the standards of care. In the UK, there is a trend towards casual work in the care sector to ensure 24 hour, 7 day a week cover, especially among large providers.

Childcare workers in publicly run childcare centres are often more secure in their jobs than those providing childcare as self-employed or through private companies. Lack of employment security is most often found in childcare workers operating from their own homes or the houses of the children they care for.

Terms and conditions

Care workers for both childcare and social care work long hours. In many countries, where care workers operate in private homes, there is a lack of supervised health and safety standards, with much lifting involved in the care of older people and of young children. There is increased pressure to complete tasks quickly with resulting health and safety risks.

Care work is considered to be mentally and physically stressful. Nursing home workers who have to lift and turn patients often develop back injuries. Childcare workers also suffer from musco-skeletal disorders as a result of lifting children. Childcare workers are also exposed to lots of children's infectious diseases. Where they lack paid sick leave this leads to presenteeism, when they have to work when ill or lose pay.

A Labour Force Survey in the UK found that 10% of social care workers, which includes social and probation workers, had a work limiting disability, which is above average for women workers (Simon et al., 2003). In addition, 7% of childcare workers have a work limiting disability (Simon et al., 2003).

Job security

The impact of social welfare policy changes, particularly the introduction of direct payments made to those needing care, is affecting the organization and status of care workers. There are some significant variations from country to country in Europe (Ungerson, 2003). These can be seen in terms of how care work is developing as a career. Perceptions of care work as a worth-while career can also develop from a more micro-level before seeing how workers are able to influence their daily work and achieve satisfaction with work tasks.

In countries where older people can purchase services themselves, the creation of new professional categories is beginning to influence the status of care work. In Germany, where a new professional category of social care worker was created at the same time as care insurance was introduced, there has been an expansion of registered care workers (Jenson, 2002). In the Netherlands, a similar process is taking place.

In some countries, a more structured and regulated care worker labour market develops when private and non-governmental agencies provide care services. Care users access these care providers through agencies. In France, Ungerson (2003) found that care workers were engaged in "multiple care relationships," often visiting up to 13 clients a day. Many had a basic qualification, which had provided them with access to training and an ability to reflect on their work.

This made them aware of the boundaries and some of the contradictions between the different tasks that they undertook. They were involved in a wide range of tasks, including cooking and shopping. The significance of these care workers being able to reflect on their work and what it means for their clients may be important for the future development of care work as an occupation (Ungerson, 2003).

A study of workplace privatization in Sweden, where private companies now run care homes, shows inconsistent findings in relation to how care workers are able to influence their work. In some cases privatization has improved the workplace atmosphere; in others it has increased insecurities and anxieties among workers. In some cases privatization has shortened the decision making process and introduced a simpler management structure. Workers often then feel that they have more power to influence their own work and to act on their own initiative (Savolainen, 2004).

In Denmark, changes in the home help services have taken place since the late 1970s, characterized by the introduction of 24 hour care which involved both home help workers and home nurses (Lewinter,

2004). As this arrangement became more established, home help workers moved from working from their own homes, to becoming part of a "semi-autonomous group" where a group of home help workers operated as a team, divided work up and sorted out problems themselves. The municipalities in charge of these teams presented this as a form of empowerment for home care workers. The introduction of the internal market and the contracting of services by municipalities are also influencing the way in which home help services are organized and delivered.

Different occupational models for childcare and out-of-school care influence to what extent there is a defined career. The type of training needed to enter the sector and the provision for in-service training and maintaining skills also influences the perceptions of childcare work as a career (Cameron et al., 2003). In childcare in Europe, the move towards integrating childcare with out-of-school care and schools is leading to increased professionalization of the workforce.

However, Cohen et al. (2004) argue that in countries where there is large private sector provision in the childcare sector the scope to transform childcare workers into a professional group is limited due to the resources and investment needed to achieve this.

Training

Training for the care of older people is less extensive than for child care workers in many countries. In most countries, care workers for older people have limited training. In some European countries there are moves towards increased training of social care workers as a way of upgrading the work, and as such improving recruitment and retention. This training is often less accessible for migrant workers. In the Unite Kingdom, training for social care is based on competency training, and this type of training is expanding, although the rapid turnover of the social care workforce means that take-up is often limited. In France, there is a more formal system of training, and many social care workers now have a qualification (Ungerson, 2003).

Childcare workers often have a higher initial level of training than care workers working with older people, although sometimes this only involved two years of training after the age of 16 or 18. A three-year training at higher education level is becoming the norm for childcare and early years workers in Nordic countries. The core 'early childhood' worker in Spain also has this level of training. In other countries, training for childcare workers is at a lower level (Cameron et al, 2004).

In the United Kingdom, Cameron et al, 2004 found that at least half of all childcare staff in the United Kingdom did not have specialist training for the job. These include child minders, many childcare staff in private nurseries, some play-workers and nannies.

In the Nordic countries the situation is different. In Denmark, the status of professional childcare is high, and training and job prospects are good. There is also a higher proportion of men working in the sector. Among family day carers, while not required to have a qualification, over 75% have a childminder certificate or have received 50-100 hours mandatory training from municipal employers (Cameron et al., 2003).

In many European countries funding for in-service training is often decentralized to municipalities, for example in Sweden, Finland, Netherlands, and Italy. In Denmark and Belgium funding for in-service training is decentralised to schools. In the United States there is a requirement at state level that childcare centre workers spend a certain number of hours per year in in-service training. Opportunities for further training in childcare are available in Spain, Denmark and Hungary (Cameron et al.,2003).

The recruitment of migrant labour can also result in a form of exploitation in relation to skilled labour, which devalues the skills of migrant workers who have trained as nurses abroad. "Both private homes and NHS trusts may obtain work permits to employ nurses, but nurses who have received their training abroad are usually subject to a probationary period to "upgrade" on the job, during which they are paid as care assistants".

Once they have completed this adaptation, which usually takes 3-6 months they can register with the Nursing and Midwifery Council, have the right to practice as nurses and be paid on the nursing pay scale. The employer is responsible for declaring that the nurses have completed their "adaptation" but "there is a financial incentive for the home to delay registration, continuing to pay on a lower scale". Nurses often borrow money to travel to the UK.The lower rate of pay restricts their ability to repay the loan (Anderson, Rogaly, 2005).

Trade unions

With the majority of care workers part time and low paid, unionization is limited in many countries because care home owners often do not recognise trade unions and also make it difficult for workers to have contacts with trade unions. Care workers employed in domestic settings also find it more difficult to organise themselves into trade unions because they are scattered and do not have the opportunity to meet other home care workers. The growing use of migrant labour in Europe and

North America also makes unionization difficult because workers with insecure residency are often afraid to access trade union support.

A Finnish trade union survey of Swedish privatization found that participation in trade union activity has also become more difficult (Savolainen, 2004). In some companies, employees have lost the right to criticize their workplaces.

In the United Kingdom, in a survey in 1997, two-thirds of care homes surveyed did not have any trade union members and did not recognize trade unions for bargaining purposes (Centre for Public Services, 1997). In Canada, unionized workers feel more satisfied with levels of pay then non-unionized workers (Canada Home care survey).

In Sweden, trade unions have played a significant role in integrating the childcare workforce through integrating their own trade unions and so strengthening their bargaining power (Cohen et al., 2004). This will also contribute to further developments of the childcare profession.

The processes of liberalization have affected the socio-economic security of care workers. The security of many childcare workers is stronger than for many social care workers. The prospects for improvements in the childcare workforce appear to be better because of the links between care and education for children. In social care, there is not the same force for change, even though new categories of social care workers are developing in some countries as a result of older people being able to purchase their own care. More widely, social care in residential and home settings is poorly paid and undervalued. Workers often have little training. The level of unionization is low.

Changing access to services

Considering how the changes in financing, organization and delivery of services have affected both access to services and the quality of services needs to seen in the context of how social welfare policies have developed in the twentieth century. In most countries there are significant differences in the ways in which childcare and care for older people have evolved as public services.

Childcare has developed in response to the growing participation of women in the paid labour force. In Europe, this should be seen in the context of the EU Employment Strategy which aims to expand the workforce. It is increasingly recognised that to expand the proportion of women in the workforce requires some form of childcare provision. Government policies differ as to which sector should provide child care even if there are government subsidies through tax rebates or child care

care vouchers and credits. The recognition of the UN rights of the child have also put pressure on governments to guarantee childcare as a social right.

Care of older people often has its origins in legislation to relieve poverty and social and social assistance (Anttonen, 2001). Defining and maintaining older people's rights to good quality social care has been a much greater struggle to achieve. The introduction of cash payments and cash transfers is considered one of the few recent examples of the expansion of welfare state programmes (Daly and Lewis, 2000). The attitude of societies towards older people is a significant barrier to improving services. The effect of commercialization of social care has often not led to improved services and research is beginning to show that access is often restricted.

Ungerson argues that the new financing arrangements that enable individuals to pay for their own care are creating a new context for care, but that the impact on the nature of the care relationship has still to emerge. The increased targeting of programmes has an effect on the distribution of care. Increased targeting of services to those with high levels of need also leads to those who have lower levels of dependency and need (especially older people) receiving fewer or even no services. The income level of an older person often determines whether additional services are paid for or whether family members take on some caring tasks.

Studies examining changes in the provision of home based services to older people in Sweden have found that since 1990, there has been a decline in the number of people receiving services, with service provision often focused on the most frail, older people. The impact of a decline in the number of beds for older people in the healthcare sector has led to more frail older people being looked after by municipal services at home. Resources are then limited to personal and home nursing care rather than municipal provision of services for shopping, cleaning, laundry and walks (Trydefard, 2003).

The needs assessment process necessary to make an individual eligible for care has been implemented more strictly resulting in people with minor needs being excluded from access to social care. This results in family members being drawn in as care providers, or for those on higher incomes using paid carers. Szebehely (2004) found that changes in home help arrangements in Sweden resulted in an increase in informal care by frail older people with lower education levels, and an increase in private care by frail older people with higher education levels.

Lewinter (2004) examined the changes in levels of provision of home care in Denmark to older people over 67, and found an increase in the percentage of people on low levels of care (< 2 hours a week) and the highest levels of care whereas these on intermediate levels (2-8 hours a week) had decreased. Trydefard, Thorslund (2001) also found that there was a wide range of variation of the level of home care available at municipal level.

As Sweden has moved toward assisted housing, this is seen administratively as a type of housing, rather than care, and so older people have to pay rent and charges for different services which are means-tested.

Ungerson (2003) found that the payment of kin to do tasks that were previously seen as part of "unpaid work" could lead to changes in family and household relations. Where a care worker is a resident member of the family, payments will contribute to the family income. But if the care worker is non-resident, commodified kin relations are more likely. In Italy, the payment for care was often used to subsidize a low income by continuing to use family and relatives to provide informal care.

In the United Kingdom there have been several trends in service provision that have directly affected users of services. With the Community Care Act of 1990 and the introduction of standards for care homes, the costs of meeting national care standards for residential homes led to both local authorities and private providers closing residential care homes with a decline in provision. By 2003, 88% of residential care had been transferred to the private sector and 66% of local authority funded home care was provided by the private sector in the United Kingdom.

This has been accompanied by a focus on home care, which provides support for people to remain in their own homes or in sheltered housing provision. Care is provided in these facilities through home care agencies. Several home care agencies, both public and private, may provide care to residents in these sheltered housing facilities as well as to users in their own homes.

Home care services show varying levels of quality. A recent survey of social workers in the United Kingdom (Centre for Public Services, 2004) found that employers felt unable to commission suitable packages of care for service users because they had to use agencies that they were not happy with, or were constrained by budget restrictions. The increase in the number of social care providers has led to more fragmented services rather than 'joined-up' service provision.

The impact of cost cutting and making social care workers do more tasks in a limited period of time has an effect on the quality of care delivered. Land (2003) gives an example of how savings on insurance may mean that a social care worker is no longer covered by an agency's insurance to take a client in a wheelchair to shops or the park. This directly affects the quality of the older person's live.

The Social Services Inspectorate in the United Kingdom compared a local authority service with that provided by the private sector. It concluded that although there was evidence of good services, they also heard about "domiciliary care, which was not providing good quality service. This was almost always in relation to independent agencies. We heard about high staff turnover, unreliability, poor training and failure to stay the full time" (SSI quoted in Land, 2003). This shows how the socio-economic security of social care workers, in relation to pay and training, has a direct influence on the quality of services delivered.

Changes in the way in which social care is financed are having an impact on how users access care and the quality of care. In Sweden and Denmark, the targeting of care towards frail older people is resulting in less dependent older people losing access to public social care services. This impacts differently on low and high income groups creating a demand for informal carers in low income groups.

Care payments have affected family relationships in both positive and negative ways. In the United Kingdom, there are early signs that the high costs of home care may result in a long term move towards institutional care for people with disabilities. This needs to be seen in the context of the long term prospects for community care for older people and whether higher costs will lead to a return to institutional provision.

Future regulatory role of government

Regulation of home care provision is perhaps more difficult than residential provision. In many countries, some form of licence is required to set up a nursing home but there are rarely any registration requirements for home care services. This makes entry into the home care market easier for new private sector providers.

There seem to be two issues that regulation has to address in the future. The first issue is how to protect the child or older person receiving care, and to assess whether the care is appropriate and delivered in a sensitive, timely manner. Second, how to protect workers delivering care to children or older people from poor working conditions, low wages and poor or no benefits. Systems of regulation for services and labour have to be able to deal with the often small scale, domestic settings in which care is delivered.

The increased participation of the private sector as a provider of care makes crucial new, more effective systems of regulation. There are different approaches to regulating the private sector, which range from a central government regulatory agency that inspects services, most often delivered in residential homes or settings, to locally arranged inspection processes.

In the United Kingdom, social care inspection agencies visit residential homes and make reports publicly available. Private sector providers are often enthusiastic about being regulated in the same way as public sector providers because they feel it makes them considered as equals to the public sector. However the scale of the task of inspecting hundreds of care homes is large, and annual inspections do not always convey how services are delivered on a daily basis. The problems of setting up adequate regulatory systems apply to both childcare and care of older people.

The nature of the relationship between government, national or local, and private sector providers plays an important role in regulation. Ayres and Braithwaite (1992) developed a concept of "responsive regulation", arguing that the regulatory strategies of government intervention should respond to the behaviour of companies, and should take into account the fact that companies sometimes seek to shape regulation to their own ends. This necessitates governments developing a better understanding of how companies operate, and the type of strategies they are developing.

The evidence of private company behaviour in the social care sector seems to show that the private sector views social care and child care as short-term investments. However the demographic changes in many countries with a growing ageing population will contribute to growing demands for services. The form in which these services will be delivered is still uncertain.

Conclusion

Changes in the provision of care for both children and older people over the past two decades have been strongly influenced by financial and demographic factors. An increasing older population, the expected reduction in the size of the tax-paying population, the expansion of women in the paid labour force, and limits on government spending, have all influenced care policies.

Public subsidisation of childcare is becoming more widely accepted by national governments. In some countries, childcare is seen as a universal service or a basic right for a child. Childcare is also acknowledged to have both caring and educative elements. This is in contrast to funding for services for the care of older people, which is influenced by the fear of escalating costs with an emphasis on ways of reducing public spending (Daly and Lewis, 2000).

Care services are provided by a range of agencies and sectors, often strongly influenced by the historical patterns of provision especially in relation to whether services are universal or targeted. Different forms of funding also exert an influence on the types of care services and the demand for care workers. The growing use of cash benefits is also shaping how services are delivered and by whom (Yeadle and Ungerson, 2002). It is also leading to different levels of take-up and so creating differing levels of access to services for older people.

Provision by non-public providers has been encouraged in almost all European countries whatever the underlying forms of provision, although family provision of care is still important. The proportions of private provision vary widely from country to country. For example, in Germany and the Netherlands, families as well as the voluntary sector provide services. In the United Kingdom, the family and the private sector are dominant care providers (Rostgaard, 2002). However, a public role in provision is still maintained in many countries even if there is a move away from direct provision to role of commissioner and regulator.

Evidence of the effectiveness of new systems of regulation is limited. Increasing homecare services require new ways of ensuring high quality standards of both service provision and workers rights.

Just as social care and childcare have only recently been researched together, so public policies need to consider care work within a single framework. Care workers are mainly women, often poorly paid, with little formal training. The future for paid social care workers lies in developing an understanding of the implications of an increasing demand for care and an apparently decreasing supply of labour in high income countries. It also involves developing a better understanding of how the needs of older people could be met through a better trained and a more highly skilled workforce.

There is a growing body of evidence that the health and well-being of older people is enhanced through increased social and intellectual activity (WHO, 2002). Caring for older people needs to involve these activities, in the same way as childcare now combines caring and pedagogic elements. Care workers will need increased and continuing training to do this. As a greater proportion of the population becomes older, the need to link care with education may also become clearer, for both care workers and receivers of care.

REFERENCES

Alber J. (1995) A framework for the comparative study of social services *Journal of European Social Policy* 5(2):131-149

Allen S.F. (2003) Working parents with young children: cross-national comparisons of policies and programmes in three countries *International Journal of Social Welfare* 12:261-273

Anderson B. and Rogaly B. (2005) *Forced Labour and Migration in the UK* Study prepared by Compass in collaboration with the Trades Union Congress

Anttonen A. (2001) The politics of social care in Finland: Child and elder care in transition in Daly M.(ed) (2001) *Care Work The quest for security* Geneva: International Labour Office

Ayres I. and Braithwaite J. (1992) *Responsive Regulation: Transcending the Deregulation debate* (New York: Oxford University Press)

Betelson P. (2003) Personal interview with Capio Chairman Per Betelson, February 2003

Cameron C. (2003) *Care work in Europe: quality employment?* Paper presented at the SARE 2003 "Caring has a cost: the costs and benefits of caring" Emakunde

Cameron C., Candappa M., McQuail S., Mooney A., Moss P., Petrie P.(2003) The Workforce Early Years and Childcare International Evidence Project/October 2003 London: Department of Education and Skills

Centre for Public Services (1997) *Undervalued work, underpaid women – women's employment in care homes* Report commissioned by the Fawcett Society

Centre for Public Services (2004) *Modernising Public Services? Evidence from the frontline Sheffield:* Centre for Public Services.

Cohen B., Moss P., Petrie P., and Wallace J. (2004) A New Deal for Children Reforming education and care in England, Scotland and Sweden Bristol: The Policy Press

Daly M. and Lewis J. (2000) The concept of social care and the analysis of contemporary welfare states *British Journal of Sociology* 51(2): 281-298

Daly M.(ed) (2001) *Care Work The quest for security* Geneva International Labour Office

Esping-Andersen G. (1990) The three worlds of welfare capitalism Cambridge:Polity Press

European Public Health Alliance EPHA (2004) Study on legal implications of services directive www.epha.org

European Public Health Alliance EPHA (2004) Briefing note to members – services, health and the internal market www.epha.org

European Union (1992) Treaty of European Union (Maastricht Treaty) www.europa.eu.int

European Union (1993) Green Book on Social Policy www.europa.eu.int

European Union (1997) European Employment Strategy http://europa.eu.int/comm/employment_social/employment_strategy/index_en.htm #ees

European Union (2004) Services in the internal market COM(2004) Draft services directive

48 Social care policies

Go K. (1998) The introduction of market mechanisms for long term care services –
an international comparison with implications for Japan NLI Research
Institute www.nli-research.co.jp/eng/resea/life/li9804.html

Holden C. (2002) *Actors and motives in the internationalisation of privately provided
welfare services: a research agenda* Paper presented at the 5th GASPP seminar,
Dubrovnik, September 2002

Jenson J. (2002) 'Paying for Caring The Gendering Consequences of European
Care Allowances for the Frail Elderly' in Women's Work is Never Done
Comparative Studies in *Caregiving, Employment and Social Policy Reform*
(ed.) S.Bashevkin New York: Routledge, 2002

Johansson S. and Moss P. (ed) (2004) Work with elderly people A case study of
Sweden, Spain and England with additional material from Hungary Care
work in Europe *Current understandings and future directions* London: Institute
of Education

Korintus M. and Moss P.(2004) Work with young children: a case study of
Denmark, Hungary and Spain Care work in Europe *Current understandings
and future directions* London: Institute of Education

Kofman E. (2004) *Gendered migrations, livelihoods and entitlements in the European
Union* Paper prepared for UNRISD submission to Beijing +10

Laing W. and Buisson (2003) *Care of Elderly People Market Survey* 2003 London

Laing W.and Buisson (2003) *Community Care Market News* November 2003

Land H. (2003) *Leaving Care to the Market and the Courts* Paper presented at the
ESPAnet Conference Changing European Societies – The Role for Social
Policy 13-15 November 2003

Lewinter M. (2004) Developments in home help for elderly people in Denmark:
the changing concept of home and institution International Journal of
Social Welfare 13:89-96

Lloyd-Sherlock P. (ed.) (2004) *Living Longer. Ageing, Development and Social
Protection* London: Zed Books

Office for National Statistics ONS (2003) Provision for children under five years of
age in England January 2003 London DFES

Pollock A (2004) *NHS plc The Privatisation of Our Health Care* London: Verso

Player S. and Pollock A.M. (2001) Long-term care: from public responsibility to
private good *Critical Social Policy* 21(2):231-255

Public Sector Privatisation Research Unit (PSPRU) (1997) *Privatisation of Care
Services across Europe* Paper prepared for the European Federation of Public
Service Unions (EPSU) London: PSPRU

Robson E. (2004) Hidden Child Workers: Young Carers in Zimbabwe *Antipode*
227-248

Rostgaard T. (2002) Caring for Children and Older People in Europe – A
Comparison of European Policies and Practices *Policy Studies* 23(1):51-68

Simon A., Owen C., Moss P., and Cameron C. (2003) *Mapping the Care Workforce:
Supporting joined up thinking* Secondary analysis of the Labour Force Survey
for childcare and social work A study for the Department of Health
London: Institute of Education

Savolainen S. (2004) A review of experiences of public services privatisation in

Sweden Finland: KTV

Szebehely M. (2004) *Home help and the Nordic welfare states.* Paper presented at the Scientific Programme for the 17th Nordic Congress of Gerontology, Stockholm, May 23-26, 2004

Trydefard G-B, Thorslund M. (2001) Inequality in the welfare state? Local variation in the care of the elderly – the case of Sweden *International Journal of Social Welfare* 10:174-184.

Trydefard G-B (2003) *Swedish Care Reforms in the 1990s and their consequences for the Elderly.* Paper presented to STAKES, Finland.

European Integration, the Open Method of Coordination and the Future of European Health Policy

Thomas Gerlinger

Health policy in the European Union today is largely shaped in national arenas. Despite certain effects of the Single European Market and rulings of the European Court of Justice (ECJ), the process of European integration has changed little in this respect. Now, however, the open method of coordination (OMC) is to establish a new regulatory approach that should allow growing supranational influence on health policy.

This article is not about the trends of national health care policies in Europe. Rather, it explores the relation that this mode of regulation creates between national and supranational levels of action on health policy and inquires into the consequences it is likely to have on national health policy in Europe.

1. Health Policy in Europe – A Domain of the Nation-States

European integration has thus far had little impact on national health policy. One of the reasons is that European institutions are subject to the principle of subsidiarity when exercising their authority in areas of social policy and elsewhere. The EU is permitted only to promote cooperation between the Member States and complement their policies.

Due to this narrowly defined scope of action the EU has explicit legislative powers in only a few spheres of preventive policy. By contrast, the authority to fashion the health care system lies entirely with the

Member States (Article 152, par. 5). They are therefore individually responsible for :

■ the type and extent of coverage afforded by the social security net in case of illness (i.e., the financing of payments and the scope of services);

■ the organization of the health care system, including the institutional structures and the division of labour between the occupational groups;

■ and the decision on the distribution of authority over the regulation of the health care systems.

In Europe at the beginning 21st century, the policy field of health – like other areas of social policy – remains mostly a national affair. Although national health-care reforms since the 1980s have often resorted to similar instruments of regulation, and although certain trends of convergence are therefore identifiable, they are not due to an establishment of transnational regulatory authority.

These reforms and trends are mainly a response to shared root conditions of economic and financial policy, to comparable health problems, and in many cases to similar kinds of shortcomings in the various systems for providing medical services. Such convergence notwithstanding, the wide range of health care systems persists, with serious differences in the structure of medical services and funding and in the regulatory framework.

Nevertheless, it would be a distortion to assert that the autonomy of the Member States is wholly unimpeded where health policy is concerned. The European process of integration has indeed gained importance for health policy in the EU Member States over the years and in some ways has generated standards for national policy. This growth in supranational influence occurs in a number of ways.

By creating and deepening the political union the EU spelled out and successively broadened the authority and obligations of its institutions to act on health matters. The treaty obliges them to direct their attention to improving the health of the population and to ensure a high level of health protection in all fields of Community policy (Art. 152, par. 1). Since the 1990s, a number of programs empowering EU institutions to protect public health have been launched by the EU Commission on the basis of its competencies in guarding against disease.

Since the second half of the 1980s, EU institutions have been assigned explicit regulatory authority in some fields relevant to prevention policy. The cardinal ones are health and safety at work and diverse aspects of health-related consumer protection, notably food safety. In these areas the EU sets minimum supranational standards that the Member States must meet.

The creation of a single European market checks the freedom of the Member States to manage their own health policies. Several decisions handed down by the European Court of Justice (ECJ) have made it plain that, although the Member States are responsible for structuring their health care systems, they must comply with the four freedoms of the single market, particularly the cross-border entitlement to health services. The ECJ's stance has substantially strengthened the rights of insured persons and providers, and has added to the refund liability of the financial carriers.

The obligation to keep the four freedoms in mind somewhat curtails the latitude for shaping national regulatory systems. Tension has arisen, for example, between European competition law and national legislation, especially where the regulation of the health care system is involved. The German system is a good example. It is moot, whether collective contracts, which are central to it, are compatible with the proscription of agreements that prevent, restrict, or distort competition within the common market (Art. 81, EC Treaty) and on the "abuse of a dominant position within the common market" (Art. 82, EC Treaty).

A declaration by the ECJ that collective health insurance contracts violate the Treaty on European Union could void key elements of the regulatory system in German health policy. Although rulings of the European Court of Justice have not indicated that the collective contract system (permitted under German health insurance law) will be classified as incompatible with European market law, there is obviously a trend towards a transnationalization of governance becoming noticeable in health policy.

2. The "Lisbon Strategy of Competition" and OMC

The process of European integration is largely influenced, if not determined, by the establishment of the Euro financial regime (with the growth and stability pact and the function of the European Central Bank at its core).

In view of the increasing economic difficulties the EU emphasized competition policy as a new path to integration – an idea that is systematically expressed in the vision formulated at the European summit in Lisbon 2000. The overriding objective is to make the EU "the most competitive and dynamic knowledge-based economy in the world". For the European Council, achieving this goal means having to:

■ consolidate public finances on a lasting basis,

■ accelerate the integration of underemployed population groups into the labour market,

■ and "modernise" (as it is called) the systems of social protection in the EU.

The Lisbon redirection of competition policy engenders economic, fiscal, and employment policy standards and imperatives that radiate into neighboring policy fields, including health. Health policy is gaining considerable importance because it is seen as having an immediate bearing on the success of the new integration strategy.

Under pressure from the targets set by the growth and stability pact, the nation-states are trying to extend strict budget discipline to their public health care systems as well. Additionally, cultivating the health of human resources is expected to help build the potential for productivity, just as encouraging the expansion of European health management is expected to build employment potential.

Both intentions are parts of a policy of fiscal consolidation. The emerging field of European health policy thus derives its developmental energy from this nexus of fiscal, competition, and employment policy.

This shift fundamentally alters the socioeconomic and political conditions surrounding health policy in Europe. In this context social policy, specifically health policy, is rising in status and is refocusing. Their new strategic appreciation is apparent in their systematic integration into European economic and growth policy: the functional objective of social and health policy has been redefined. Redistribution, the compensation of social risk, and the other classical goals are no longer the primary criteria – the main thrust now is to take the European model of development and steer it toward competition as effectively as possible.

OMC is pivotal in this reassessment and realignment of European social and health policy. Agreement on the application of this procedure is closely related to the strategic reorientation of the European integration process. It should improve voluntary cooperation and the transfer of sound procedures between the EU Member States, helping them to continue development of their national policies. The salient point is to increase the efficiency with which the national policies in the various policy fields are integrated into efforts to achieve the overall strategic goal. This is greater competitiveness of a European knowledge-based economy by consolidating public budgets and modernizing social protection.

OMC was defined for the first time in the conclusions drawn by the Council of Lisbon. It encompasses the following core elements:

■ The setting of guidelines for the development of individual policy areas, including a timetable for the realization of short-, medium-, and long-term objectives

■ The establishment of quantitative and qualitative indicators and benchmarks to ease comparison of national practices and to identify sound processes

■ The adoption of European guidelines in the policies of the Member States through development of concrete objectives and the enactment of appropriate measures

■ The regular supervision, evaluation, and mutual examination of the measures taken and the progress achieved

As defined at the Lisbon summit, OMC differs overall from past policy strategies and procedural practice in distinct ways that mark it as a new regulatory model.

OMC is a procedure for developing common policies that goes beyond the traditional rule- and norm-setting established in the Treaty on European Union – that is, beyond predominantly issuing guidelines and regulations. The idea is to foster political commonalities between the Member States, not by transferring resources of control (e.g., rights and money) but rather by advancing a process of coordination and learning ("soft regulation") that leaves the formal authority of the Member States intact.

The European Council, the European Commission, and the EU Council of Ministers become the foremost actors of European-wide coordination. The key role lies with the European Council, which is explicitly accorded a strengthened managing and coordinating function. It is responsible for supervising the implementation of the strategies and processes and for taking corrective action if necessary.

The purpose is to promote political commonalities between the Member States by engaging in the desired joint process of coordination and learning, which tends to rely on voluntary coordination, on communicative and interactive forms of control and dispenses with binding targets and formal sanctions.

OMC thus takes a kind of "third way", leading between the classical quest of harmonization on the one hand and mere recommendations or intergovernmental agreements on the other. This process tries to inaugurate the transition from a strategy of harmonising institutions to a strategy of harmonising policy objectives. Convergent developmental processes are to be achieved through an EU-wide coordination of policy formulation, without formally jeopardising national sovereignty. OMC therefore links two contrasting interests: that of EU institutions in broadening their influence on health policy and that of the Member States in preserving their sovereignty.

In addition to employment policy, provision for old age, and measures against "poverty and social exclusion", OMC shall be applied to health policy. In several reports and other documents passed by the EU since the Lisbon summit the European Commission and the European Council describe the problems that the health care systems of the Member States have in common and define EU-wide goals for reform of the systems for providing health services. Challenges that health policies in Europe share and must address are

■ the rise in the ratio of old people to the total population,

■ the impacts of new technologies and therapies on medicine,

■ and the mounting popular demand for medical care and appropriate services as living standards and levels of education improve.

The Commission noted that these matters raise the question of budget management and escalate the pressure to curb costs. It is therefore necessary to develop "clear, transparent and effective evaluation mechanisms". Thereby, the European Commission unequivocally makes the long-term financial viability of health policy a regulatory premise of economic and fiscal policy in the EU.

The Commission formulates three main objectives of health policy in the EU to be achieved simultaneously:

■ The establishment of universal access to high-quality health care.

■ An increase in the transparency and quality of the health care systems by evaluating medical procedures and service structures.

■ Continuation of reforms aimed at cost containment (flanked by endeavors to consolidate public budgets and ensure adequate funding for health care).

In view of this analysis and set of goals, the EU concludes that the health care systems of the Member States must be adapted to meet the demands of a dynamic, growth-oriented economy. In the Council's view, the changes must involve not only cutting costs but also modernization of the systems in order to foster their efficiency. This message is still the tenor of the Commission's analyses and proposals for action.

3. OMC's Likely Impact on Health Policy

There are indications that OMC widens opportunities to coordinate national health policies. However, it also has likely practical difficulties and risks for the delivery of health care.

3.1 Problems Specific to the Field of Health Policy

Research is increasingly identifying the limits and troublesome aspects of benchmarking and best practice approaches. These problems are especially serious in the evaluation of health care systems. Health care systems are complex economic sectors or systems of social action centered on rendering personal services. The staple regulatory instruments (e.g., forms of compensation and institutional arrangements of medical service providers) operate within the context of a specific system or in interaction with other elements of it.

In addition, there are problems resulting from the social complexity of health as a "good". Services provided through health policy relate to the treatment of diseases, the promotion of health, or both. Health and illness are the result of an almost overwhelming number of variables, which, moreover, occur in different combinations from one case to the next. In most cases, the utility of certain interventions can be reliably judged only after a long period, if at all.

Given the heterogeneity of the health care system and the societal complexity of health as a phenomenon, it is hard to imagine how a benchmarking process is supposed to identify examples of best practice that could prove to be universal standards for providing effective and efficient services. Compounding this problem is the undeniable fact that definitions of indicators and benchmarks always reflect individual interests and power relations.

If nothing else, this conundrum demands data of exceptionally high quality on which to base health policy. The existence of that quality cannot be taken for granted, at least not yet. Dissimilar national data-gathering methods and differing statistical and conceptual distinctions in the individual countries of the EU seriously restrict even rough comparisons of resources and their use in EU Member States. Limitations on the measurement of health care outcomes are far greater still. Even where such comparative data exist, it is difficult for the ascertained outcomes of health care measures to be causally attributed to discrete features of the systems under which those measures were administered.

3.2 Conflicts over policy-related goals

But the main problems for the implementation of OMC will probably arise from the menacing goal conflicts that could ensue from utilizing the health policy and health policy targets of the European Council and European Commission for purposes of competition policy and the consolidation of public budgets. The objective of ensuring a high level of social protection and open access to services of the health care system implies a high level of public spending, which would clash with the cost-cutting necessary to achieve the Maastricht stability criteria and would thus weaken the EU.

Conversely, the intended utilization of health policy to further competition policy and cost containment can encourage privatization of medical treatment, endangering the goal of ensuring a high level of social protection and unhindered access to health care services.

But if the implicit or explicit goals are not achievable all at once and if goal conflicts are foreseeable, then the political decision-makers setting the agenda for health policy will eventually have to rank priorities in health policy.

Because the calculation of the annual public debt includes both the state health systems and quasi-governmental social insurance institutions under public law, it is not surprising that the financial development of the health systems is monitored in view of its potential to jeopardise fiscal stability.

This strategic logic for anchoring the coordination of health policy firmly in the European financial regime's targets for stability explains why the policy goals of consolidation can be expected to have priority over those of medical services. By the same token, cost containment may well take priority over the goal of ensuring comprehensive, high-quality care when it comes to setting indicators and benchmarks.

The European Commission's report about the future of the health care system and care for the aged consistently points towards prioritization of this kind. It emphasizes that health policy "is vital for the implementation of quality and viability strategies, which must respect the principles laid down in the Broad Economic Policy Guidelines for 2001.

Health policy thereby comes to center on the premises of economic policy designed to consolidate public budgets and stabilize prices and on the accumulation of physical and human resources in the private sector. Accordingly, it appears absolutely logical that cost containment be given preference over the goal of ensuring comprehensive, high-quality care in the setting of indicators and benchmarks.

Recent experience supports this expectation. A few weeks ago, in March 2005 at the Brussels summit, against the background of the economic crisis and increasing rates of unemployment the European Commission and the European Council reformulated the Lisbon Strategy.

The renewed "Lisbon strategy" re-emphasizes the focus on growth and employment. The European Council instructed the Commission to develop integrated guidelines for the period between 2005 and 2008.

These guidelines will be valid for three years and shall be implemented into national reform programs to be presented by the Member States in autumn 2005. In those programs the nation states are supposed to say precisely what measures they intend to take in order to support the policy of growth. All aspects relevant for the Lisbon Strategy, including health policy, shall be integrated into one report. The connection between health policy and economic policy is now even drawn closer

Priorities like these would tie European health policy into trends that have existed from some time at the national level. Since the 1980s, cost containment and consolidation have been acquiring ever greater standing as a "fiscal imperative" of government policy goals in the field of health within the developed capitalist democracies. In the 1990s, the specter of economic stagnation and the pressure resulting from the steady climb in the costs of national health care systems only fueled this trend, worsening the conditions for funding innovative forms of care and threatening to cement social barriers blocking recourse to services. The longer the ensuing scarcity of funding for the health system persists, the more likely it is that there will be trouble with policy on medical services.

3.3 OMC as an accelerator of reform

One conceivable way of deescalating this conflict between the policy goals of fiscal consolidation and those of improving medical services is to pursue reform policies that would develop the existing potential for thrift and efficiency in the national heath care systems. This approach would be fully compatible with the goals of coordinating health policy at the European level and could address structural shortcomings. The use of OMC could help enhance the chances of prevailing over such defects and defeating obstacles to innovation. Systematic collection and comparative analysis of information about the individual health care systems when preparing benchmarking reports could lower the transaction costs of gathering information, could simplify the recognition of flaws, and could thereby better the conditions necessary for broad learning effects. OMC could definitely help speed up reform by functioning mainly as a clearinghouse for information. As we will come to know in this conference, the health care systems of the Member States offer many suitable opportunities for such accelerated efforts to modernize.

Again, Germany is a good example. In German health policy and among scientific experts, there is broad consensus that the system of statutory health insurance in Germany suffers from a dearth of efficiency and quality. Compared to other systems in the world, it combines high expense and only mediocre health results. Structural weaknesses of the medical service system are blamed for the most part, especially the lack of preventive health policy, the marked segregation of the medical service sectors, and an overreliance on specialist services. Defying every attempt at reform, these structural drawbacks in the German health care system are exceedingly stubborn. If international comparison were to intensify awareness of, for example, the segregation between out-patient and in-patient care or the high representation of specialists in outpatient medical services, it could facilitate public discussion and criticism and help create a public climate conducive to reforming and overcoming these deficiencies. In this way, pressure could grow to change structures identified as inefficient or suboptimal and adapt them to superior models.

4. Conclusions

In principle, it appears to be possible that OMC can help streamline the supply structures in the health care system in the EU Member States in a way that lowers the pressure to ration health services. However, the contextual conditions and strategic bearings of initiatives coming from the EU and finding their way into national health policies through OMC give reason for great skepticism:

First, the EU's political elites are not inclined to embark on the contentious and risky path of calling challenging mighty vested interests, particularly on matters of health policy. The preferred road to success in the international competition to attract industry is to retract the social security net and accentuate "personal responsibility."

Second, strengthening the European level of action in health policy does not eliminate those alignments of national forces and contextual conditions that have already thwarted or hampered modernization of medical care structures in the Member States, not least in Germany.

The functional embedding of OMC in a specific vision of competition policy, the obligation of EU Member States to adopt the provisions of the European Economic and Monetary Union, and the policy-related regulatory and control problems specific to the health sector feed the concern that using OMC in the field of health policy could eventually degrade social protection when illness strikes.

Therefore, it is wholly probable, that the outlined changes in the different arenas of Europe's multilevel system will turn out to be policy-field-specific components of a process that has been described as a transition to a new European social model.

Embedded in the European financial regime and the revamping of competition policy along the lines of the Lisbon strategy, a new vision is beginning to surface in health policy and other fields. In the traditional European social model social policy was understood as an expression of public responsibility for the social welfare of the population. The new vision now replaces "government interventionism in the interest of social policy" with "government interventionism in the interest of competition policy" (Aust et al. 2002).

If it succeeds the foremost goal of strategies for active social policy would no longer be to correct adverse economic and social distributional effects of the market and to ensure protection against the social risks of life. It would be replaced by the goal of adapting the European model of development to the exigencies of competition in a transnationalized economy and of using social and health policies primarily as resources for increasing productivity and competition. Against this background, increasing pressure on unhindered access to high-quality health care has to be awaited. Against this background, increasing pressure on unhindered access to high-quality health care has to be awaited.

References

Aust, A./Leitner, S./Lessenich, S. (2002): Konjunktur und Krise des Europäischen Sozialmodells. Ein Beitrag zur politischen Präexplanationsdiagnostik, in: Politische Vierteljahresschrift, Vol. 43., No. 2, pp. 272-301

Busse, R./Wismar, M./Berman, P.C. (eds.) (2002): The European Union and Health Services. The Impact of the Single European Market on Member States, Amsterdam

de la Porte, C./Pochet, P. (2002): Building Social Europe through the Open Method of Co-ordination. Brussels

Freeman, R./Moran, M. (2000): Reforming Health Care in Europe, in: West European Politics, Vol. 23, No. 2, pp. 35-58

Gerlinger, T./Urban, H.-J. (2004): Auf neuen Wegen zu neuen Zielen? Die Offene Methode der Koordinierung und die Zukunft der Gesundheitspolitik in

Europa, in: Kaelble, H./Schmid, G. (eds.), Das europäische Sozialmodell. Auf dem Weg zum transnationalen Sozialstaat (WZB-Jahrbuch 2004), Berlin, pp. 263-288

Hodson, D./Maher, I. (2001): The Open Method as a New Mode of Governance: The Case of Soft Economic Policy Co-ordination, in: Journal of Common Market Studies, Vol. 39, No. 4, pp. 719-746

Jorens, Yves (ed.) (2003): Open Method of Coordination. Objectives of European Health Care Policy. Baden-Baden

Radaelli, C.M. (2003): The Open Method of Coordination: A New Governance Architecture for the European Union – Preliminary Report – Stockholm

Schmucker, R. (2003): Europäischer Binnenmarkt und nationale Gesundheitspolitik. Zu den Auswirkungen der "vier Freiheiten" auf die Gesundheitssysteme der EU-Mitgliedsländer, in: Jahrbuch für Kritische Medizin, No. 38: Gesundheitsreformen – internationale Erfahrungen. Hamburg, pp. 107-120

Schulte, B. (2002): Die "Methode der offenen Koordinierung". Eine politische Strategie in der europäischen Sozialpolitik auch für den Bereich des sozialen Schutzes, in: Zeitschrift für Sozialreform, Vol. 48, No. 1, pp. 1-28

Food and Health Safety in the United States and the European Union

Dr. Philip van Meurs and Dr. Lila Antonopoulou

Introduction

It is safe to say that in almost every textbook about political science in general, a part is devoted to lobbies and interest groups. These, often informal, groups play an important role in influencing policymaking[1]. This is nothing special. It is almost unavoidable that not only the individual citizen but more so interest groups, be they citizens' initiatives, industrial or farming organizations, present their concerns and interests to lawmakers and government officials. Often their share of the economy, and therefore also of the economic and financial well-being of the individual citizen, is very large.

If the interests of industry or farmers are not taken sufficiently into account, then economic well-being, in the form of sufficient available jobs and income but also the safety and reliability of consumer products, is at stake. Also research and the willingness to contribute to public projects and regulations concerning the specific sectors of the various interest groups may be endangered. However, if the argument of economic interest takes the upper hand, other aspects of a product may become less important. Problems with safety, consumer health and pollution, among others can and often will be ignored.

It suffices to point to the record of the United States in relation to the Kyoto protocol. Under pressure of powerful industrial lobbies the United States government will not propose the Kyoto protocol for ratification in Congress. The issue is not that there is a risk that Congress will not ratify it, although they may well not ratify the treaty, but that the US government believes that the Kyoto protocol takes away economic advantages enjoyed by United States business. The argument that the Precautionary Principle adopted in the protocol is not scientifically sound is merely a smokescreen.

Powerful lobbies and interest groups that are well organised often have a much greater influence on policy making than public opinion[2]. Lobbyists, interest groups and political action committees (PACs) influence policy making in the US:

(1) through campaign contributions and other material contributions;

(2) through the development of expertise and sharing this expertise strategically with policy makers; and

(3) by ensuring that those who get elected are in favour of their viewpoints, interests and policies.

The sharing of expertise gives the Interest Groups, lobbyists and PACs the function of service bureaux[3]. The total operating costs in the US can be conservatively estimated at $12 billion per year.

The United States has a unique system with regard to lobbying, in that the political parties (only two – Republicans and Democrats) are not cohesive parties like in Europe but merely an aggregate of relatively independent factions. They come under attention, and govern only 'spasmodically'. Their legislators do not have to toe the party line, because they are not worried about attaining a cohesive majority to control government or influence the date of new elections, like in parliamentary democracies. If US parties would do that it can be assumed that the influence of interest groups or lobbies would probably be much smaller[4].

Before we speak about interest groups it is necessary to say what they are. We believe that the definition of interest groups from Wright is useful. According to him a political interest group, or organized interest group, is:

"a collection of individuals or a group of individuals linked together by professional circumstance, or by common political, economic, or social interests, that meets the following requirements: (1) its name does not appear on an election ballot (no political party); (2) it uses some portion of its collective resources to try and influence decisions made by the legislative, executive, or judicial branches of national, state, or local governments (no hobby groups or incidental groups that do not allocate resources to influencing); and (3) it is organized externally to the institution of government that it seeks to influence (no coalitions of government officials that seek to influence their own institutions, like congressional groups like for instance 'the Congressional Black Caucus', etc.)."[5]

One of the basic types of political interest groups certainly concerns corporations. They have become very influential, since they feel that the political climate has moved away from big business since the 70s. Therefore a more vigorous representation of corporate interests was deemed necessary.

What is true for the United States is to a certain extent true for the European Union, where lobbies also play an important role. The farmers' lobby, for instance, is powerful enough to slow down and disrupt decision making and reform in the field of the Common Agricultural Policy (CAP). In doing so the farmers' lobby imperils the formation of an economically and financially sound budget for the EU.

The example of the farmers' lobby shows that also on a Union level the EU and its institutions are a target for interest groups and lobbies. Instead of PACs one speaks of Eurogroups because these are interest groups that present themselves on a European rather than on a national level. This is not to say that national interest groups are not present. Other interests are represented by large business firms who have established offices in Brussels alongside other interest groups.[6]

Like in the US, interest groups serve as service bureaux. But there is a difference with the US: on a national as well as on a Union level, government and political parties use their own research institutions and expertise. The influence of lobbies is difficult to determine. They provide information and try to persuade policy makers of their causes. It is much more difficult to influence nominations since, for key posts, this is in the hands of the Commission and the council of ministers. The governments of the member states have a considerable say in this. On the national level there is usually an institutional involvement of the classical interest groups, the unions and the employers' organisations, as well as government.

In general, lobbies and interest groups find it almost impossible to approach the European Council or the Council of Ministers, since meetings are not public. These councils exist as a discussion and decision institution for national interests. They do not present themselves as a collective entity. Only the president in office (a regulating position among the member states) may invite an important interest group for consultations.[7]

The Commission often makes itself available to interest groups for two reasons. The first is that the Commission wants to understand what interests and opinions exist in the field of its policy proposals, and gain specialised knowledge of these groups. Secondly it wants to use powerful and/or important interest groups as a demonstration that important actors in the field support a certain policy proposal.[8]

Like in the United States, but presumably on a lesser scale, the EU experiences the influence of lobbies and interest groups. One can argue that the influence of interest groups and lobbies enhances the democratic process, because those involved can have their say through policy makers or officials. It is often argued that one of the main aspects of democracy is that the citizens both as individuals and collectively can legitimately pursue and defend their own interests without anyone telling them what this interest is.[9]

Furthermore they may persuade policy making away from the public will. The public will is, of course, not well defined. But it can be perceived in an often subterranean discontent. In the EU signs for this can be perceived in the emergence of populist and sometimes radical nationalist political groups and parties. In the US this can be seen in the general disinterest of the public in policy-making, and often distrust of the Federal Government. In general the complicated political processes in both the US and the EU, with the influence of interest groups and 'big business', as the public perceives it, do not create an atmosphere of trust for the average citizen.

The United States and the European Union are not readily comparable in many respects, but they are both major economic players in the world economy. At least in economic sense their relative power is in the same order of magnitude. Therefore they are the objects of research in this paper.

We will discuss the approach of the United States and the European Union concerning food safety, the environment, and the influence of many lobbies and interest groups. We can largely generate the approach from the conflicts that exist between the United States and the European Union. And apart from the influence of specific interest groups we will see that there is a growing fundamental methodological difference between the two trade partners concerning safety. This difference partly centres on the acceptance and rejection of the precautionary principle.

The Precautionary Principle is attacked by many, notably interested parties like farmer organisations and the bio-industry, on the grounds that it is 'not scientific'. They plead for the elimination of this principle from government considerations and decisions, especially in the European Union.

The Center for Trade Policy Issues, in an article concerning Genetically Modified Organisms (GMOs) states:

> "The EU has banned all foods containing GMOs on the basis of the "precautionary principle," under which regulators do not need to show scientifically that a biotech crop is unsafe before banning it; they need show only that it has not been proved harmless. Jettisoning scientific risk assessment and replacing it with a precautionary approach will open the entire trading system to interruptions based on arbitrary justifications. Capricious labelling requirements will also proliferate. Such labels are unjustifiably stigmatizing and costly and offer no consumer health or safety benefits."[10]

Moreover they expect that scientific progress will slow when the precautionary principle is allowed to prevail [11]. Let us look for a moment at the elements of the precautionary principle versus and in conjunction with risk analysis.

The Precautionary Principle and its Enemies

The principles of prevention and of precaution are closely related. Because they are so closely related they often get mixed up in the political debate, especially where policies of prevention and protection of goods such as public health or the environment are concerned. [12]

Granted that the precautionary principle is, per definition, of a preventive character both in its content and aims, this mixing up is partly understandable given the extremely wide field of applicability of the principle of prevention. In fact the latter principle includes the former, irrespective of whether preventive measures are or are not precautionary measures.

What then is the criterion that allows a valid distinction to be drawn between the two? The answer is that the preventive principle helps guide the authorities in the adoption of measures deemed necessary both for preventing a predicted and imminent risk and for limiting damage. Prediction is made possible by scientific inquiries and practices, which produce evidence of a causal link between an element or state of affairs and apparent injurious effects. In other words, the prevention principle allows the adoption of public measures with a view to minimising the impact of an already identified risk. Therefore methods of risk assessment and risk management belong to the preventive principle, since they base themselves on scientific evidence concerning the risks involved. [13]

Despite heavy reliance on scientific knowledge there are a growing number of cases in which the present level of scientific knowledge makes it impossible positively to identify the existence of risk and thus makes the prescribing of preventative measures impossible. In such cases one must initially proceed with caution[14]. Nevertheless, the precautionary principle is the very principle that allows state regulation to transcend simple prevention, based on scientific conjecture regarding impending risk, and organise itself upon the adoption of measures against possible risk whose nature or origin remain uncertain or even unknown.

Contrary to the more traditional principle of prevention invoked on the basis of hard scientific data, the precautionary principle is invoked when no scientific evidence or even agreement among the scientific community exists. In this sense it is possible to characterise the precautionary principle to begin with as a policy instrument allowing authorities to respond, even though the causes of the crisis remain unknown. Such a principle would then facilitate and authorise the adoption of preventive measures against certain human activities, even though no scientific evidence is available to determine whether or not these activities pose risks for human health.

Two approaches are immediately called for regarding the 'core' of the precautionary principle. The first concerns the so-called 'technocratic' approach as regards the scope of the implementation of the precautionary principle. Risks and injuries from human activities can be reduced to a 'cost problem' which can be dealt with by application of quantitative methods [15]. Does the technocratic approach cover merely the existence of risk, injury, and impending damages which, for the authorities, would be the decisive factor in the taking of precautionary measures against a specific activity?

One answer to this question runs as follows [16]:

When there is a strong likelihood of impending risk or damage it is sufficient to implement the preventive principle, and whichever measures such principle dictates.

When strong likelihood of impending risk is combined with the seriousness of the damage that may be inflicted, again there is no need for the precautionary principle since the two sides of this 'uncertainty' – impending risk and serious damage – are subject to scientific inquiry and knowledge even in relative terms.

The implementation of the precautionary principle depends, prior to any other consideration, on the uncertainty attending the sense of impending risk; in such cases it is evident that the more uncertain the impending risk/damage, the more the uncertainty predominates regarding the seriousness of such state of affairs.

Finally, since scientific uncertainty does not refer to the degree of seriousness of risk, forecasts about impending risk allow only for taking measures under the title of 'precautionary measures'. The precautionary principle comes into effect when it is not possible for policy makers to assess risk and damage.

The second approach, although connected with uncertainty, leads back to the 'source' of the precautionary measures taken by the authorities. Previous decisions were made in similar circumstances under conditions of scientific uncertainty, conditions that involve chance and risk. The element of uncertainty regarding impending risk is, indeed, immanent in decisions and activities in which the agent is engaged and which involve risk; the essence of this uncertainty lies in that present decisions made assessing such activities which aim to provide protection for agents, do not rule out future 'negative results' (harm or damage) and indeed results such as one sought to preclude in coming to those initial decisions.[17]

Moving from the level of the individual to a wider social realm, and subsequently to that of the civil authorities, it can finally be ascertained that uncertainty as an immanent element of precautionary measures is the reverse side of the uncertainty that subsists in risk-laden human decisions.

That is to say, faced with the possibility of a negative outcome issuing from decisions made about activities involving risk, and therefore faced with the possibility of catastrophic consequences of which one was initially uncertain, the societal body erects a series of measures or decisions (precautionary measures) to avert such consequences – depending on the very same uncertainty which attended the risk-laden decisions.

General Principles of Food Safety Policies

We have discussed the precautionary principle above. The European Union has largely adopted this principle as a safeguard in the absence of scientific information[18]. Furthermore the EU and its member states take an active role in ensuring that no harmful effects will come from the introduction of GMOs.[19]

The American Food and Drug Administration together with its counterpart for meat, poultry, and egg products, the Food Safety and Inspection Service (FSIS), has adopted general scientific standards for evaluating the safety of food in the United States. These are generally:

■ The method of risk assessment and

■ The precautionary approach.

The heading 'risk assessment' contains also risk management and risk communication. The methods concerned are briefly described above under our discussion of the precautionary principle. The precautionary approach however, needs some elaboration.

Precautionary Approach

The FDA does not intend to introduce the precautionary principle. The precautionary approach is rather different, in that it is directed at preventing the introduction of harmful substances in food or food products.

The genesis of many health, safety, and environmental laws is associated with the prevention of undesirable events and the protection of public health and the environment. Specific prevention and protection measures reflect differing provisions of law, regulation, and circumstances. However, they all are risk-based. The precautionary approach is exercised in a variety of ways.

An example of the U.S. precautionary approach to risk is the control system for ingredients in food and feed, such as the prohibition of feeding certain animal proteins to ruminants to prevent the introduction of BSE in this country. In implementing this prohibition through a regulation, the government followed the existing APA (Administrative Procedure Act) procedures to explain in the Federal Register why it is proposed to take the action, including a description of the risk, and to evaluate the comments received from industry, academia, private citizens, and government agencies before publishing its final regulation.

Another illustrative example of the precautionary approach is the pre-market approval requirements established by law for food additives, animal drugs, and pesticides. The products are not allowed on the market unless, and until, they are shown by producers to be safe to the satisfaction of the regulatory authorities. ... the data – or the lack of data – drive a decision for approval. The evaluation of all is documented. The final decision explaining the basis for all significant conclusions is published in the Federal Register. Persons disagreeing with the decision may file an objection with the reasons for disagreeing and request a hearing. After administrative remedies for appeal are exhausted, the government may be challenged in court on its approval or denial of a petition.[20]

In other words the precautionary approach is a product of risk assessment. Another term for it is the above discussed Preventive Principle.

The bones of content

There are basically two areas where the US and the EU have a different approach concerning food safety. These differences have led to trade conflicts. In their turn these conflicts have been dealt with in the World Trade Organization, but this did not lead to a solution. The basis of the conflicts is that the European Union in principle does not want to import foodstuffs that are either enhanced in quality and quantity through the use of (growth) hormones and/or are changed in their genetic make-up. It is clear that the closing of the European markets constitutes a great loss for the agricultural sectors in the US and Canada (which applies basically the same policies as the USA) and other countries like Brazil, and also for the industries behind the research in genetically modified organisms.

The continuous EU bans on these products have resulted in a trade war where the US and Canada have imposed sanctions on EU products exported to North America. The use of sanctions has gone back and forth. It is safe to say that in spite of the importance of the arguments for and against the different approaches to food safety, these sanctions are not good for the relations between the USA and the EU in particular or for world trade in general.

Hormone Beef

The web-site of Friends of the Earth, an US environmental organisation, mentions that since the 1970s the United States meat industry has used hormones in order to stimulate the growth of animals[21]. What they should mention as well is that also in Europe farmers have used hormones for the same purposes. In 1981 the European Community restricted the use of hormones in meat, and an import ban on hormone treated meat and meat products has also been in place. This ban has resulted in protests by the United States and ongoing negotiations within first GATT (General Agreement on Tariffs and Trade) the forerunner of the WTO (World Trade Organisation) and later in the WTO itself.

It should be mentioned, however, that the hormones that stimulate growth are normally produced naturally in the animal. Three of the hormones used to influence growth in animals, estradiol, progesterone and testosterone, are naturally occurring hormones produced by all humans and food animals. Three other hormones that are used as well are trenbolone acetate, zeranol and melengestrol acetate (MGA). They are synthetic hormones: trenbolone acetate mimics testosterone, zeranol mimics estradiol, and MGA mimics progesterone.[22] Three natural hormones are used and three synthetic ones that have the same effect as the three natural hormones. The question is, of course, whether hormone treated meat is safe for human consumption?

Another organisation the Codex Alimentarius Commission (short CODEX), set up in 1963 jointly by the Food and Agricultural Organisation and the World Health Organisation, has developed standards pertaining to the use of hormones in meat production[23]. The 1995 food standards adopted by the Codex allow a certain level of hormone residue in meat seen as not dangerous for health.

> "[R]esidues arising from the use of testosterone and oestradiol-17B as a growth promoter in accordance with good animal husbandry practice are unlikely to pose a hazard to human health and that the amount of exogenous progesterone ingested in meat from treated animals would not be capable of exerting an hormonal effect, and therefore, any toxic effect, in human beings."[24]

The Codex Commission even goes to the position that the establishment of an ADI (Acceptable Daily Intake) and an MRL (Maximum Residue Limit) for certain hormones used in meat production is not necessary. [25]

The adoption of these standards is seen by many as controversial, especially because the standard allowing the use of hormones in meat won by only 4 votes (33 in favour and 29 against, 7 abstentions). Interestingly this vote replaced an earlier one that was against the use of hormones in meat. It is said that the United States used its influence in order to sway the vote in favour of the use of hormones.[26]

This political game, denounced by many environmental groups, is nothing out of the ordinary in international negotiations. Every actor, country or organisation, pursues what it sees at its national best interest. Not only the United States but also the European Union, its member states, and many other countries all over the world, try to turn policies of international organisations like the United Nations and its agencies in their favour.

In the United States the situation is transparent insofar as the companies that lobby the US government are well known. Companies involved in the production of hormones used in meat production but also in the genetically modification of crops and animals for agricultural use have a paramount interest in a favourable international climate in relation to their activities. Therefore they try to influence the United States government. They are part of one of the strongest lobbies in the

US. One could say that lobbying is the result of the possibilities of a democratic system, where not merely the voters can support policies or parties that support their interest but also other legal entities like interest groups or companies.

Clearly it should not be assumed, before judicially valid proof is obtained that demonstrates otherwise, that companies involved in biotechnology deliberately put the health of consumers at risk. However, as we have seen with the problems of the Kyoto protocol, it may be that the line between consumer health and economic advantage is approached here. The approach to food safety is consistent with the so-called 'scientific approach'. Various studies, including studies done by the European Union (the Lamming report) show that the health risks of consumption of hormone treated beef are very low. Risk analysis shows that the hormone treated meat has hormone residues far below the level of acceptable daily intake (ADI). The problems with the EU are not about the validity per se of these studies, but about the limits of the scientific instruments used in risk analysis. Another problem concerning consumer health is that it is difficult to research long-term health risks, since there are no valid scientific instruments to do so.

The position of the United States on the hormone meat issue involves a mixture of scientific and legal objections.

Central is the question concerning the certainty of scientific finding concerning the use of hormones in meat. The United States argues that by the highest scientific standards the use of hormones is safe. This is confirmed by studies in the European Union itself. The problem, however, is that these studies do not involve the study of long term effects of the intake of low level residue hormones by the consumer. As we have said above, such a study is difficult to perform, and there are also moral problems with a long term study.

Feeding people, by means of an experiment, residual quantities of animal hormones in their diet is not very ethical, since people are not guinea pigs. The only viable study of the long term effects of the consumption of hormone treated meat would be a study of the whole of the US population. The problem there is that a relatively clean experiment cannot be done because of various other food related influences could disturb the outcome of such a study (which would be so in any population: the US would be interesting since many people consume hormone treated meat).

The arguments of the United States against the prohibition of hormone treated meat in the European Union can be summarised as:

European Union research shows that hormones in beef do not pose a risk (this is research done on the basis of risk assessment by the Lamming Group).[27]

The prohibition of hormone treated meat is illegal under the SPS agreement since there is no sufficient scientific evidence that meat treated with the six hormones allowed in the United States is harmful to the health of the consumers.

It cannot be justified as a provisional measure, i.e. awaiting further research. The ban imposed by the European Union is permanent.

The prohibition is trade restrictive, i.e. it is used to favour trading parties (EU farmers) and discriminate others (US farmers) where similar conditions prevail. [28] This means that the United States claims that the argument of possible health dangers through the consumption of hormone treated meat evades the real issue, namely EU protectionism.

The prohibition is arbitrary and unjustifiable since it imposes different measures in different situations.[29]

According to the WTO-Appellate Body the burden of proof lies with the actor who imposes measures. In this case the European Union has the burden of proof. Moreover proof has to be given according to the methods of risk assessment.

> "We note that in this dispute the European Community, which has the burden of proving that it based its measures on a risk assessment, has not provided any evidence that the studies it referred to (in so far as they can be considered as part of a risk assessment) or the scientific conclusions reached therein, have actually been taken into account by the competent EC institutions either when it enacted these measures (in 1981 and 1988) or at any later point in time. We note, in this respect, that none of the preambles to the EC measures at issue mention any of the scientific studies referred to by the European Community. These preambles only refer to the non-scientific reports and opinions of the European Parliament and the EC Economic and Social Committee, which cannot be considered as part of a risk assessment."[30]

The Appellate Body in its conclusion reversed this requirement of the SPS agreement. The Appellate Panel also allowed the precautionary principle as a health protection principle in accordance with the SPS agreement.[31]

Genetically Modified Organisms

Another issue concerns genetically modified organisms (GMOs). For many consumers and consumer organisations there are many problems with GMOs. These problems occur partly because much is unknown about the side effects of the introduction of these organisms in the environment and in food. The FAO (Food and Agricultural Organisation of the United Nations) has summarised these concerns in a number of key issues for ethical consideration:

Food safety.

The foundation of consumers' concern about GMOs is food safety.

Because of experiences with non-GMO food problems such as allergens, pesticide residues, microbiological contaminants and, most recently, bovine spongiform encephalopathy ("mad cow" disease) and its human counterparts, consumers are sometimes wary of the safety of foods produced with new technologies. The approaches being taken by governments to ensure the safety of GMOs are discussed in the sections under risk analysis.

Environmental impact.

The potential of GMOs to upset the balance of nature is another concern of the public. GMOs are "novel" products which, when released, may cause ecosystems to adjust, perhaps in unintended ways. There is also concern about the possibility that genetic "pollution" will result from crossing with wild populations. As with non-GMOs, an issue is whether pre-release testing (especially when limited to laboratories or computer models) is an adequate safeguard for the environment or whether post-release monitoring is also necessary. The extent of post-release monitoring needed to protect ecosystems, especially with long-lived species such as forest trees, becomes an ethical as well as a technical issue. The current understanding of the environmental impact of GMOs is reviewed in the relevant chapter.

Perceived risks and benefits.

In forming their views about GMOs, consumers weigh the perceived benefits of accepting a new technology against the perceived risks. Since practically none of the currently available or forthcoming plant and animal GMOs presents obvious benefits to consumers, they question why they should assume possible risks. It is said that consumers take the risks while the producers (or the suppliers or companies) reap the benefits. The science-based methods used to assess risks, together with their relationships with risk management and risk communication, are discussed in the chapter GMOs and human health.

Transparency.

Consumers have a legitimate interest in and right to information with regard to GMOs in agriculture. This begins with rules for the transparent sharing of relevant information and the communication of associated risks. Science-based risk analysis seeks to enable experts to make decisions that minimize the probability of hazards in the food supply system and the environment. Consumers, however, may also wish for more transparency to protect their right to exercise informed consent on their own. An often-discussed set of means intended to protect these rights is the labelling of products, whether or not they are derived from GMOs. Informed consent and labelling are also discussed in the chapter GMOs and human health.

Accountability.

Consumers may wish to be more involved in local, national and international debates and in policy guidance. At present, there are very few fora available to the public to discuss the wide range of issues relating to GMOs. A shortage of fora can, understandably, lead to advocates concerned with one aspect of GMOs, such as environmental impact, pushing their concerns into a forum set up for another aspect, such as labelling. A related issue is how to bring the private sector transparently into public fora and, subsequently, how to hold public and private sector agencies accountable.

Equity.

So far, the development of GMOs in agriculture has mainly been oriented towards cost-reduction at the farm level, primarily in developed countries. Societies have ethical standards that acknowledge the importance of ensuring that those who cannot satisfy their basic food needs receive adequate means to do so. Ethical analysis can consider the moral responsibility of societies, communities and individuals to ensure that economic growth does not lead to an ever widening gap between the poor majority and the wealthy few. When appropriately integrated with other technologies for the production of food, other agricultural products and services, GMOs may, among other biotechnologies, offer significant potential for assisting in meeting the human population's needs in the future. An ethically salient issue that then emerges is how the development and use of GMOs in agriculture can be oriented towards improving the nutrition and health of economically poor consumers, especially in developing countries.[32]

These are issues shared by many consumers in the EU and find their expression in the numerous environmental organisations but also in the concerns expressed regularly in the European media.

Notwithstanding these issues, in the field of GMOs the European Union does not impose an outright ban on products coming from genetically modified organisms. On the contrary there is concern in the EU that Europe may lag behind in the development of knowledge and products using biotechnology. This is demonstrated in a quote from the European Commission:

> "In Europe and elsewhere, intensive public debate has emerged. While the public debate has contributed to awareness and concrete improvements on important issues, it has also focused narrowly on genetically modified organisms (GMOs) and specific ethical questions, on which public opinion has become polarised. In the Community, like in other regions and countries, the scientific and technological progress in these areas raises difficult policy issues and complex regulatory challenges. Uncertainty about societal acceptance has helped to detract attention in Europe from the factors that determine our capacity for innovation and technology development and uptake. This has stifled our competitive position, weakened our research capability and could limit our policy options in the longer term."[33]

This shows that the position of the European Commission is less restrictive than on hormone treated meat. However, there is no agreement on whether such products pose a danger to human and animal health or to the environment.

In the United States this discussion is also not yet a thing of the past. GMOs, especially the variations developed by various companies, are grown more and more. Although the Food and Drug Administration, the US food quality-testing agency, tells us these crops are not only safe for consumer health but also safe for the environment, not everyone agrees.

A study done by the British government shows that genetically modified crops can be harmful to the environment. Insects – not only pests but also useful insects like bees – are often the victims of the anti-pest genes inserted in the genetic make-up of crops.[34] The argument in favour of genetically modified crops that produce insecticide substances is that the use of these crops will result in a higher yield.

However, in Congress there are proposals to label food that is produced from GMOs or with the help of GMOs.[35] This shows that concerns about the safety, but also about citizens' right to know what they are consuming is taken seriously by US legislators.

The European Union has demanded too, that products that contain GMOs are properly and clearly labelled, so that at least the consumer can decide whether he or she wants this product or not, on the basis of the information on the label.[36] The EU labelling regulation has been challenged by the United States on the ground that, among other things, it restricts trade. The United States brought the EU before the dispute settlement body of the World Trade Organisation in May 2003.

The objections of the United States against the current EU regulation concerning the labelling of GM produced foodstuffs are the following:

■ The use of genetically modified organisms is safe under the SPS agreement. We have already seen that the methods of scientific testing are limited to risk analysis. The precautionary principle is seen as non-scientific.[37]

■ Labelling imposes trade barriers against US products on technical grounds. Article 2 of "The Agreement On Technical Barriers To Trade" state that technical regulations shall not impair equal treatment of products (i.e. domestic in relation to imported products). Article 5 states that like products should be treated in the same way in all circumstances. (xxx) The EU and the US disagree about the definition of 'like products' in relation to genetically modified organisms, i.e. crops in relation to non-modified ones.

■ A request by the United States for consultations was granted but the consultations did not result in agreement. It seems that the problem that the United States has with restrictions and labelling by the European union is not so much with the measures themselves but the effect that these measures have on other countries in the world that are potential importers or actual importers of US agricultural products.

The wariness of the Europeans in regard to US agricultural products may find agreement in other countries, especially Asiatic countries like, for instance, China which form enormous potential markets.

The requirements for allowing Genetically Modified Organisms in the environment and the food chain

We will now look at the requirements of both the Federal Agencies of the USA (FDA and Department of Health and Human Services) and the European Union (European Parliament, Commission and the Community Reference Laboratory (CRL)).

Decision making for both sides is somewhat different. In the EU the European Parliament has together with the Council of Ministers, issued a directive concerning "the deliberate release into the environment of genetically modifies organisms"[39]. This high level statement shows clearly that not only the European citizens are concerned with this issue, but also the EU in its high level organs as well as its member states represented in the Council of Ministers.

The Department of Health and Human Services with its Food and Drug Administration has a more independent role from Congress. This is certainly not to say that in the USA there is less concern or interest in the introduction and use of genetically modified organisms, but that the decision making system is different from that in Europe. That there is another attitude towards these issues in food safety is already shown in the issues concerning hormone treated meat. This shows also in the issues around the introduction of GMOs.

Food quality requirements in the United States

The broad regulations under which the FDA works is the Act on Food and Drugs[40]. The Act regulates liabilities and requirements. However, it supplies a framework in which hormone treatment and biotechnology can get an interpretation, but only in jurisprudence. The act itself does not mention these elements specifically.

Under the act:

> "the FDA is responsible for ensuring that all foods in the American food supply conform to the applicable provisions of the law. The act provides FDA with broad authority to regulate the safety and wholesomeness of food. In particular, the act prohibits the adulteration of food under section 402 of the act (21 U.S.C. 342) and the misbranding of food under section 403 of the act (21 U.S.C. 343). The act also requires that all food additives (as defined by section 201(s) of the act (21 U.S.C. 321(s)) be approved by FDA before

they are marketed (sections 409 and 402 of the act (21 U.S.C. 348(a) and 342(a)(2)(C)). FDA is authorized to seek sanctions against foods that do not adhere to the act's standards, through seizure of foods that violate the act under section 304 of the act (21 U.S.C. 334); the agency is also authorized to seek an injunction against, or criminal prosecution of, those responsible for introducing such foods into commerce under sections 302 and 303 of the act (21 U.S.C. 332 and 333)".[41] In the proposed FDA rules of 2001 the duty of showing that a genetically modified component of food (or animal feed) is safe and wholesome lies entirely with the producer. The FDA will not itself start an investigation or scientific research. The producer or vendor of food containing GMOs has total responsibility. If anything goes wrong the producer/vendor can be sued for damages. There are certain administrative requirements such as a Premarket Biotechnology Notice that has to be submitted at least 120 days before a certain food stuff is marketed[42]. The FDA will allow or prohibit a certain product on the basis of this notice.

One could assume that given the strong reliance on scientific data certain materials, organic or inorganic, that have been proven harmful or poisonous, are actively banned from human food, but that other materials, like certain hormones at certain levels or genetically modified organisms constituting food products wholly or partially, are allowed since their harmfulness is not proven. This seems to be unscientific itself. The precautionary principle prevents this from happening. Foodstuffs are allowed when it is scientifically proven that they are not in themselves harmful.

Food Quality in the European Union

Among the Commissioners in the European Commission there is a special Commissioner for Health and Consumer Protection. Food safety is included in his portfolio [43]. In Europe the counterpart of the US FDA is the European Food Safety Authority (EFSA) established under the overall responsibility of the Directorate General for Health and Consumer Protection.

As in economic and monetary matters the Commission has the power to act for the whole of the European Union.

DG Health and Consumer Protection and its agency

The European Food Safety Authority coordinate research and provide the commission with advice and recommendations. The Authority is relatively young. It was officially set up at January 28, 2002. The legal framework is laid down in the joint European Parliament and Council regulation (EC) No 178/2002, 28/01/2002).

The principles for food safety in the European Union are laid down in the White Paper on Food Safety.[44] The approach to food safety is integral. The White Paper states that:

"Following the Commission's Green Paper on food law (COM (97)176 final), and subsequent consultations, a new legal framework will be proposed. This will cover the whole of the food chain, including animal feed production, establish a high level of consumer health protection and clearly attribute primary responsibility for safe food production to industry, producers and suppliers. Appropriate official controls at both national and European level will be established. The ability to trace products through the whole food chain will be a key issue.

"The use of scientific advice will underpin Food Safety policy, whilst the precautionary principle will be used where appropriate. The ability to take rapid, effective, safeguard measures in response to health emergencies throughout the food chain will be an important element." [45]

Three areas of concern are Food Safety Controls, Consumer Information and relations with producers outside the EU.

The principles of Food Safety in the EU are:

An integrated approach. This is clarified by the term 'Farm to Table'. Therefore the different aspects of food safety, i.e. "scientific advice, data collection and analysis, regulatory and control aspects as well as consumer information, must form a seamless whole to achieve this integrated approach."[46]

The role of the participants concerning food-safety must be clear. Farmers and other producers have a primary responsibility.[47] There are several authorities that will monitor their behaviour and are able to enforce required standards. The Commission coordinates the activities of the national authorities so that the integrated approach is guaranteed throughout the EU.

All foodstuffs and their ingredients must be traceable to their origin.

The procedures applied to food safety must be transparent. This means, among other things, that scientific opinions and measures must be made public.

The method of Risk Analysis is central in a food safety policy.

"Where appropriate, the precautionary principle will be applied in risk management decisions. The Commission intends to present a Communication on this issue." [48]

It is clear that the precautionary principle plays an important role. The Commission wants to err on the safe side, and this is the main reason for the reservation against hormone treated meat and genetically modified organisms. The Commission wants to comply with WTO standards of free trade. Therefore the regulations temporarily or permanently prohibiting certain substances apply equally to the European Union itself as well as to imports from countries outside the EU.

This approach is not without its drawbacks. The production of hormone treated meat is cheaper in relation to the quantity and quality of the product. It puts European meat production in a less advantaged position in relation to producers in countries where the use of hormones is allowed. However scientific uncertainty, especially in respect to long term effects of the consumption of hormone treated meat, and the resistance of consumers against hormone beef, ensure that the prohibition will not be lifted very soon.

In relation to genetically modified organisms, the drawbacks of prohibition may go beyond mere production advantages. The production of GMO crops may not only be cheaper, but also friendlier to the environment in that fewer pesticides are required (the counter argument is that the anti-pest substances developed in the crop itself may be dangerous for the environment). Another element is that scientific research in the field of genetic modification of organisms will lag behind in Europe in relation to other parts of the world, notably the United States.

Nevertheless, the choice has been made in the direction of food safety security. So long as there is no decisive evidence that the concerned food stuffs or ingredients are safe the European Commission will resist attempts to bring them on the market in the EU.

Conclusion

Food safety policies in the United States are not merely directed towards consumer health, but are part of international trading strategies. The arguments are not merely about free trade and the removal of restriction in regard to 'like' products, but also about 'proving' that the possible difficulties that countries and notably the EU have raised against US products like hormone treated meat, genetically modified organisms and products made with these hormone meat and/or genetically modified organisms are irrational.

This applies especially to what in our view is an artificial difference between risk analysis and the precautionary principle.

Moreover the United States is prepared to impose heavy import duties, especially on products from the European Union in order to help to convince its trading partners to adopt the US point of view. The price that has to be paid by the US economy is a price that Washington is willing to pay, since future gains would not merely be 'free trade' for US products but also political dominance in respect of the international institutions involved and ultimately of the trading partners of the United States. This would imply that, although lobbying and hence the influence of large organisations and companies are important, there is a consistent overall policy relatively independent from these influences.

Real equality in trade matters and real free trade are only options if US interests profit directly. This is clearly demonstrated in quite a different trade conflict between the United States and the European Union, namely about steel production. If the United States respected all aspects of the principle of free trade, it would respect the WTO ruling and modernise its own steel industry. But this would have consequences for employment in US steel corporations … therefore the US will not abide by the free trade principle.

Free trade is only important if it is beneficial to the US economy. The argument that the third world may profit from it as well is only used in this respect. If third world production, which will be mostly agricultural, becomes better in quality and quantity and thus effectively competes with US products, the principle of free trade will quickly be abandoned.

In relation to the European Union there is another problem. The EU is slowly becoming a great economic power. The EU acts in the economic and trade matters as a single and competent entity, in place of its member states. This necessarily means not only a loss of sovereignty for its member states but also a loss of power for the United States, which has dominated the world economy since the Second World War.

For the European Union the issue is not challenging the power of the United States: the interest groups, especially those of consumers and environmentalists, have perhaps an even larger influence in the Commission than their American counterparts have in the US government. Ultimately, however, issues of power politics will reach the Commission. This depends for a great part on the further development of the European Union.

It seems today that US attempts to curb European power have an opposite effect in that they will push the member states of the EU closer together, making them more willing to accept a federalist approach. The trade issues concerning hormone beef and GMOs are not the only ones. The United States and the European Union have many more conflicts in this field. It is to be hoped that consumer health and safety together with just economic relations in the world remain the main consideration in these conflicts.

References

1. See a relatively old book by Robert Dahl, *Democracy in the United States-Promise and Performance*, Boston, 1981, p. 234 ff. and a relatively new book by Kay Lawson, *The Human Polity- A Comparative Introduction to Political Science*, Boston, 1999, p.133 ff.
2. John R. Wright, *Interest Groups and Congress, Lobbying, Contributions, and Influence*, New York: Longman, 2003 [1995], p.2.
3. Wright p. 8.
4. Wright, p. 14/15 and E.E. Schattschneider, *Party Government* (New York: Holt, Rinehart and Winston, 1941), p. 192
5. Wright. p. 22/23.
6. Neill Nugent, *The Government and Politics of the European Union*, London, MacMillan, 1999 [1989], p. 303.
7. Nugent p.307/8.
8. Nugent p. 310/11.
9. Robert A. Dahl, *Democracy and its Critics*, Yale University Press, New Haven and London. 1989, p.73-74.
10. Ronald Baily, *The Looming Trade War over Plant Biotechnology*, August 1, 2002, Center for Trade Policy Studies.
11. Ibid.
12. See Lila Antonoloulou and Philip van Meurs, The Precautionary Principle in the European Union, in *'Health Policy'* Volume 66, Issue 2, November 2003 , Pages 179-197.
13. The Codex MRA from the Food and Agriculture Organisation (FAO) of the United Nations, Alinorm 99/13 Appendix IV, www.foodriskclearinghouse.umd.edu/Codex_MRA.htm.
14. Vaque, Ehring and Jacquet, supra, p. 90
15. See Luhmann (1991) Soziologie des Risikos, Berlin-New York: De Gruyter, p. 19, quoted in Georgiadou (1999) *Risks in post-modernity. A socio-political analysis*, in Louloude, Georgiadou and Stavrakake (eds.) Phusis, koinonia, episteme, sten epoche ton 'trelon ageladon'. Diakindineuse ke Avevaioteta (Nature, Society, Science at the time of the 'mad cows disease'. Risks and Uncertainty), Nephele : Athens, p. 92.
16. Cameron and Abouchar, supra n. 1, p.103

17. see Luhmann, and Georgiadou, supra n.23, p.91
18. Directive 2001/18/EC of the European Parliament and of the Council of 12 March 2001, PART A, GENERAL PROVISIONS, Article 1.
19. Ibid. Article 4.
20. U.S. Food and Drug Administration, U.S. Department of Agriculture, March 3, 2000, United States Food Safety System, Chapter B. Risk Analysis And the U.S.'s Precautionary Approach
21. International web site of 'Friends of the Earth', www.foei.org/trade/activist-guide/hormone.htm p. 1, WTO, EC Measures Concerning Meat and Meat Products (Hormones), Complaint by the United States , Report of the Panel, E 26 RUSA [1], p. 10
22. www.useu.be/issues/BeefPrimer022699.html
23. www.codexalimentarius.net. There is a long history going back into the 19th century about the establishment of national and international food standards, see historical page of the FAO, www.fao.org/docrep/w9114e/W9114e03.htm.
24. WTO, EC Measures Concerning Meat and Meat Products (Hormones), Complaint by the United States , Report of the Panel, WT/DS26/R/USA, 18 August 1997 [1], p. 9
25. ibid., p.8.
26. Friends of the Earth, ibid.
27. Lamming Group, a research group set up by the European Commission in order to assess the risks of the consumption of hormone treated meat, mentioned in the complaint by the United States in WTO, EC Measures Concerning eat and Meat Products (Hormones), Complaint by the United States , Report of the Panel WT/DS26/R/USA, 18 August 1997 [1] p. 11.
28. WTO ibid., p.14.
29. ibid., p.15.
30. ibid. p. 223
31. Appellate Body, EC Measures Concerning Meat and Meat Products (Hormones), AB-1997-4, p.104-5
32. http: 'www.fao.org/DOCREP/003/X9602E/x9602eO4.htm
33. 52002DC0027 Communication from the Commission to the Council, the European Parliament, the Economic and Social Committee and the Committee of the Regions – Life sciences and biotechnology – A Strategy for Europe /* COM/2002/0027 final */ Official Journal C 055 , 02/03/2002 P. 0003 – 0032
34. NRC-Handelsblad, 17th October, 2003.
35. The Genetically Engineered Food Right to Know Act, HR 2916, Introduced July 25, 2003 in the US House of Representatives.
36. Council Directive 90/220/EEC.
37. Board on Agriculture and Natural Resources, Genetically Modified Pest-Protected Plants: Science and Regulation (2000), p. 2.
38. TBT Agreement, Articles 2 and 5.
39. Directive 2001/18 EC of the European Parliament and of the Council of 12 March 2001.

40. 21 U.S.C. 342.
41. Department of Health and Human Services, Food and Drug Administration 21 CFR Parts 192 and 592 [Docket No. 00N-1396] RIN 0910-AC15 Premarket Notice Concerning Bioengineered Foods AGENCY: Food and Drug Administration, HHS. ACTION: Proposed rule.
42. In the text concerning the proposed premarket notice concerning bioengineered food (21 U.S.C. 331, 342, 343, 348, 371) it is the producer who fills out a form to notify the FDA that genetically engineered foodstuffs or foodstuffs that contain genetically engineered substances are being put on the market. This gives the impression that, although this reporting procedure is certainly not entirely voluntary, no active controls are being exercised by the FDA. Eventual research in the dangers and/or benefits of certain foodstuffs come afterwards.
43. At the moment (December 2004) this is the Greek commissioner Markos Kyprianou.
44. Commission of the European Communities, Brussels, 12 January 2000, COM (1999) 719 final, White Paper on Food Safety
45. White Paper on Food Safety, p.3.
46. Ibid., p.8.
47. Ibid.
48. Ibid., p. 8/9.

Trade Unions and Health Promotion

Mauri Johansson

ABSTRACT: Health Promotion (HP) is still a rather new and developing concept, compared to disease prevention and cure. However, HP opens up a deeper understanding of what health is about and the broadness of the concept, including basic requirements of strong democratic structures in societies, globally, nationally and locally. Workers' unions have since the middle of the 1900 century been the leading forces in the struggle for better social and health conditions. Many basic demands have been fulfilled and enforced by law. Historically, though, the power of the working class fluctuates. Under the contemporary conditions of an aggressive global neoliberalism it seems that unions are under threat, being directly attacked and even disintegrating. Consequences of this development are hazardous for the health of workers and their families.

Experiences form the Nordic Countries since early 70s will be presented. Organising close cooperation between workers and their unions on the one hand and professionals on the other can strengthen the power of unions in HP and simultaneously induce a deeper understanding among professionals of the contexts and conditions workers are subject to.

Introduction:

Since the 19th century, workers have organised in trade unions and parties to strengthen their efforts at improving workplace health and safety, terms and conditions, working hours, wages, job contracts, and social security. Cooperation between workers and their organisations and professionals has been instrumental in improving regulation and legislation affecting workers' health.

Health promotion is rife with fundamental political, socioeconomic, philosophical, ethical, gender- and ethnicity-related, psychological, and biological problems. Analysis of power and context is crucial, focusing on political systems nationally, regionally, and globally. In the face of rapid neo-capitalist globalisation, unions represent a barricade – probably the strongest – in defence of the health and safety of workers and their allies, not only in workplaces, but in society in general.

Work, health and trade unions

Workplace health promotion (WHP) focuses on improvement of workers' health in its broadest sense: workplace community as the core of interventions. WHP may address lifestyles, early detection, workplace health hazards, and possibly wider matters such as improving quality of life and physical, psychological, and social contexts and services both at the worksite and beyond. WHP represents an "intermediate" or meso level between micro ("intrapersonal") and macro ("policy") levels of health promotion, exploiting the physical proximity and social connectedness of employees. Trade unions may play a powerful role in initiating and implementing WHP programs.

From the very beginning of the trade union movement, fundamental issues included health and safety at work, influence over job conditions, working hours, wages, stable job contracts, and social security issues. Shop stewards and safety representatives were elected to defend and improve these elementary rights; all this is included under what is today called "health promotion". In this there is inherited a strong and active democratic tradition and a continuous control and acceptance between the workers and their elected representatives, which at least in Europe is no longer usually the case between voters and their political party representatives – not even in the so called "socialist" or "social democratic" parties.

With a few outstanding early exceptions (Ramazzini, Pott, Engels), it is remarkable how late systematic research on the fundamental relations between work and health (both taken in the broadest sense) was started, including the uncovering of the role of unions. Seen from the angle of the everlasting class struggle, victories for the workers imply higher wages, more safety, and more humane treatment of the worker or the working class.

Just to mention some few examples from later times, the French Revolution in 1789 that overthrew the former power structures (feudalism) and put power in the hands of the rising bourgeoisie brought with it considerable changes both in theory and practice, e.g., creating a hospital system as we know it today and medical services based on well trained physicians where the post-revolutionary ideology opened new ways to understand illness and disease. So also the popular unrest in the early years of industrialism, in the times of Karl Marx – mid 19th century – resulted in better conditions for the working class.

In the last part of the 19th century in Germany, Reichskanzler Otto von Bismarck created several laws against the socialist organizations and unions, but at the same time passed social laws about workers' protection, compensation for injuries at work and support in case of illness. This was, without a doubt, to meet the critique from the socialists and to weaken their arguments and power.

But the real radical improvements came with the Russian revolution in 1917, which secured workers in most European countries the 8-hour workday and other fundamental rights. Also World War II, which in fact was an intercapitalist fight for the reorganization of colonies and power worldwide, resulted in basic improvements for the workers and people in general, by the creation of the United Nations and the Universal Declaration of Human Rights, combined with the funding of the World Health Organization and its well known definition of health.

The study of the distribution of diseases in populations, called epidemiology, has earlier been dominated by studies of infectious diseases, based on simple theoretical models. Not until about three decades ago was "social epidemiology" established as a modern discipline, accompanied by more comprehensive models for understanding the nature of all types of diseases and illnesses.

An appreciation of the central role of the social context, and the shift in focus from individual to family, group, collective, neighborhood, and class, opened up a deeper understanding of the very nature of illness phenomena. A recently published textbook on social epidemiology

(1) provides an excellent overview of the development of this discipline and introduces some alternative paradigms. Similarly, critical epidemiology

(2) emphasizes emancipation, interculturality and dialectical realism in the study of health and human development.

Links between trade unions and health and social scientists and practitioners in the collective improvement of workers' health and in alleviation of social inequalities in health are essential. Thus, using data from six countries, Elling (3) demonstrated how organized labor on a "macro" level forced governments and parliaments to pass laws that improved workers' conditions during the 20th century. In the Nordic countries, where well-organized unions have been active since the beginning of the 20th century, with membership rates of up to 80 to 90 percent of all workers, and covering most of the labour force, even today remarkable results are evident.

Cooperation between unions and working-class parties has been the key strategy. There are examples of cooperation between workers and their organizations, on the one hand, and scientists, practitioners of medical, social, industrial hygiene, and technical occupational health promotion, and officers in social, labor, and health administration, on the other. These coalitions have occasionally been instrumental in improving regulation and legislation affecting workers' health.

In the years following 1968, when joint activities between workers and professionals sprang up all over Europe, a local painters' union in Aarhus, Denmark, contacted a group of medical students to ask for their help in finding out about severe central nervous system symptoms among its members. Using interviews, short questionnaires, and scientific documentation, the investigation showed that exposure to organic solvents could explain both acute and chronic symptoms described by the painters. This led to a joint report (4), which demanded that working conditions be changed and the toxic substances eliminated. The cooperative endeavor resulted in a new type of organization – "Cooperation Workers – Academics" in Aarhus and "Action Group Workers – Academics" in Copenhagen – which still exist. These groups have produced more than 80 non-technical reports, pamphlets, and other materials covering a broad range of industrial and other areas of working life.

Most of the projects were initiated by single workers or shop stewards, who, with help from their local unions, investigated the problems in collaboration with active students and professionals. The publications were widely distributed among workers and used in training sessions for safety representatives. They influenced working conditions throughout the country. The "painter reports" were followed by systematic research at the university level, confirming the findings (5–7). Threshold limit values for organic solvents were reduced, and the painting industry was forced to develop and use water-based paints. Chronic illnesses among painters and others exposed to solvents were now compensated as occupational diseases – more than 3,000 cases have been compensated in Denmark during the last 25 years.

The number of new cases of chronic solvent syndrome was considerably reduced during the 1990s and today almost no new cases are seen. Strong counter-actions were taken by the chemical industry, which hired scholars to demonstrate the research was false (8). The public presentation of the oil industry report in 1984 was greeted by red union banners in the university auditorium to mark the protests.

These worker–academic reports had a considerable impact during 1972–75 in Denmark. In a state committee set up to propose revisions of the 1954 Worker Protection Act, seven of the reports were acknowledged for the way they exposed the problems (9). The committee proposed the main elements to be included in a new Working Environment Law, passed in 1975 and enforced in 1977. Workers' influence on their working environment and on occupational health and safety in general was secured. This law in many respects served as the inspiration for the E.U. Framework Directive 1989/391. Also, the Danish National Confederation of Trade Unions (LO) was forced to accelerate its working environment programs and demanded input into university research (10).

A similar worker–academic coalition has been active in Finland since the early 1970s. It has been publishing reports steadily over the years and occasionally has joined forces with the Danish organizations. This nongovernmental organization has published an 8- to 16-page newsletter four times a year, prepared and distributed pamphlets, booklets, and books, and organized various campaigns and training sessions. In particular, it prepared a set of strict threshold limit values for workplace chemicals and a draft for a law on occupational health services (OHS). Both were printed and distributed among trade unions and unionists, particularly safety representatives, and most likely influenced legislation and regulation of workplace chemical exposures and OHS in Finland.

These are a few examples from the Nordic Countries, characterizing the so called "Nordic Model", which is now under serious threat from the European Union that favors models based on law, not on agreement between employer's organizations and trade unions.

As you can see, it started with prevention. But during the past two decades or so a new term, health promotion has been introduced. The term stresses a proactive approach: instead of waiting for unwanted injuries or diseases you as a workplace health "expert" can intervene and change the working situation, so that these negative effects are avoided. This also means that the expert has the initiative and knowledge. If the expert does not carefully negotiate his plans with not only the employer, but also the workers, many mistakes can be done.

But the political influence, exercised by workers unions on the health of nations goes much beyond the workplace health conditions.

Some reflections on health, illness and disease

Health is a central precondition for optimal human flourishing. Impairments, even smaller, retard development even if they, admittedly, in case you survive, also can support, individually and in the collective, new ways of thinking and acting. But severe impairment often places burdens, both on the individual and the collective. The consequences are highly different, depending of the degree of development of the society and the actual amount of resources.

Human flourishing ("eudaimonia") in the classic Greek society was the central goal for all human development, characterized not only by absence of illness, but feelings of peace, mental and emotional balance – in reality a goal in itself. But only a small minority, the free men on the agora, were included in this inner circle – women, strangers and slaves for example were not involved.

The medical theories of those times and nearly 2 000 years ahead in Europe, USA and later on worldwide were based on theories of balance between the liquids in the body (humoral theory) and the balance between the body and the surroundings, developed by Hippocrates, Galen and their followers. Slowly, in the period of Enlightenment in the 16th century, where René Descartes presented his dualistic philosophy, the foundations of the current scientific thinking were laid.

Philosophy was gradually split up into separate sciences, where the natural sciences, especially physics, with Newton, took the leading role, showing remarkable results in the understanding of nature and the possibilities to manipulate and "conquer" it. Chemistry and biology followed later on. Medicine was eager to use the methods and techniques developed by the natural sciences, and incorporated them efficiently in its research paradigm, once again with impressive results in many areas of physiology and diseases.

But, there is a big "but": The Cartesian dualism, transplanted to medicine, resulted in a division between body and soul. The body was thought of as a complicated machine, the soul something eternally existing, separated from the body. By the successful development of laboratory sciences in medicine, anesthetics, efficient pharmaceuticals and supporting sciences like statistics and epidemiology, this biomedical way of thinking became totally dominant during the 20th century.

Medicine was more and more defined as a natural science, based on hard evidence. Diagnostics and therapy, not prevention of illness, came into focus. The body, its organs and biochemical components captured all attention. Cure, not care was the slogan. Environments, physical, chemical, psychological or social were not considered especially relevant to explore. This changed gradually the role of doctors. The humanistic, "art"-aspects of the physicians work, deteriorated. Research prioritizes pharmacotherapy and advanced medico-technical interventions – in short: activities suitable for making profit.

Disease prevention and especially health promotion lack this quality, unless specially adapted for it (like fitness centers etc.). Health now is transformed to a commodity – it is not any longer considered as a central human right.

Considerable interesting research has been recently presented (11):

> "Three fundamental discoveries of current neuroscience will forever change the way of understanding human nature. The first is that novelty, enriching life experiences, and physical exercise can activate neurogenesis – new growth in the brain – throughout our entire lifetime. The second is that such experiences can turn on gene expression within minutes throughout the brain and body to guide growth, development, and healing in ways that could only be described as miraculous in the past… The third discovery is that whenever we recall an important memory, nature opens up the possibility for us to reconstruct it on a molecular-genomic level within our brain.

> "That is, we are constantly engaging in a process of creating and reconstructing the structure of our brain and body on all levels, from mind to gene. The profound implications of these three discoveries suggest the following: (1) How we can use our consciousness to co-create ourselves; (2) New approaches to stress, psychotherapy, and healing arts; and (3) A new bridge between the arts, humanities, science and spirit.

> "These processes may however be also reversible, not only creating health and well-being, but illness and disease as well. Deprivation and extreme poverty, humiliating treatment and loss of dignity, social inequalities (racism, gender inequality), violence, torture, hopelessness, enduring stress, endless suffering etc. may cause the opposite results: degeneration of brain and body, i.e. illness and disease, psychic as well as somatic, and even sudden death" (12, 13).

Johan Galtung created the concept of "structural violence" to describe these forms of violence, used against individuals, but often even against whole populations and races.

Economic and social rights, meaning power, must be equally distributed in the processes of empowerment. Protection of the weak party is more than legal protection of civil and political rights. Luckily, critical jurists are in many countries aware of these problems and speak up.

We can speak of the terrorism of money (12). Human rights are best understood and most accurately and comprehensively grasped from the point of the poor. Farmer (2003) advocates an agenda for research and action grounded in the struggle for social and economic rights, an agenda suited to public health and medicine and whose central contributions to future progress in human rights are linked to the equitable distribution of the fruits of scientific advancement.

The concepts of action, conscientization and emancipation are clear also in the works of Freire, Lukács, Fromm, Breilh, and many others. Such an approach is in keeping with the Universal Declaration of Human Rights but runs counter to several of the reigning ideologies of public health, including those favoring efficiency over equity. A focus on health alters human rights discussions in important and underexplored ways: the right to health is perhaps the least contested social right, and a large community of health providers – from physicians to community health workers – affords a still untapped vein of enthusiasm and commitment.

This focus serves to remind that those who are sick and poor bear the brunt of human rights violations. By including social and economic rights in the struggle for human rights, we help to protect those most likely to suffer the insults of structural violence.

Some ethical reflections on health promotion

Ethical codes are not always helpful. They often share an unacknowledged agreement, that in fact all humans are NOT born equal and that this inequality accounts for both differential distributions of disease and differential standards for care. Conventional medical ethics and bioethics must be discussed. Ethics draws strength from experience-distant disciplines such as the classical philosophy.

We have to support the new branch of philosophy, the praxis-philosophy that works hand in hand with the specific sciences and arts in the context of life. Bioethics has been and continues to be a phenomenon of industrialized nations. The debate on ethical matters has been dominated by experts, not those who have far more direct experience, and emphasizes individual conceptions.

There have been few attempts to ground medical ethics in political economy, history, anthropology, sociology, and the other contextualizing disciplines.

The Canadian philosopher Charles Taylor argues that individualism and instrumental reason are the two primary sources of modern malaise, the perplexing sense of loss, decline, and disintegration felt in contemporary culture. To the extent that the pursuit of a science of health promotion reinforces – or fails to challenge – the dominant instrumental ethos, the field adds its weight to the following problems

(1) the foundations of values are being undermined;

(2) clarity about goals is being subordinated to the pursuit of more effective means;

(3) the intrinsic value of various social practices is being eroded;

(4) the relationship between means and ends misconstrued; and

(5) respect for the dignity and autonomy of individuals threatened as the intent of effect change in others' behavior is promulgated.

Buchanan's (14) proposal to avoid the negative developments in health promotion is to reorient research, training, and project activities toward strengthening people's capacity for reasoning wisely and cultivating greater mindfulness and civility; in practice that means a reintegration of means and ends.

Rather than treating people as objects for study, this means a more participatory research, a process in which people come to understand themselves better and see more clearly what ought to be undertaken to realize ends of their own choosing. Rather than instilling an ethos of technical efficiency, a reorientation of academic training programs is needed to enhance students' capacities for exercising more discerning ethical and political judgment, wherein field work would necessarily assume greater prominence.

Rather than having program objectives and methods prescribed by the results of experiments, we should break down the distinction between program developers and program recipients to the greatest extent possible, in a process in which health promoters would cast off the heavy mantle of behavior-change experts and rejoin their communities as fellow citizens.

Economic and inequity aspects on health and illness

From a growing amount of scientific documentation we already know that inequity alone causes differences in the illness distribution and preterm death. The famous Whitehall study by Michael Marmot and collaborators in U.K. demonstrates that even relative deprivation has these effects. In a recent article Marmot concludes:

"A prominent feature of health in all industrialized countries is the social gradient in health and disease. Many observers believe that this gradient is simply a matter of poor health for the disadvantaged and good health for everyone else, but this is an inadequate analysis. The Whitehall Study documented a social gradient in mortality rates, even among people who are not poor, and this pattern has been confirmed by data from the United States and elsewhere.

"The social gradient in health is influenced by such factors as social position; relative versus absolute deprivation; and control and social participation. To understand causality and generate policies to improve health, we must consider the relationship between social environment and health and especially the importance of early life experiences" (15).

Another tendency that I consider alarming is a consequence of the World Bank and IMF activities worldwide. The continuous and increasing economic blood-letting, especially in the low-income countries, has extended poverty, deterioration and privatization of public services, transference of huge amounts of money to the richest capitalist countries, producing eternal debt in several countries.

All low income countries should immediately be released from these debts. The social deterioration, with slums, unemployment, criminality, corruption, substance abuse, AIDS etc., is an obvious explanation of the declining of health status and preterm deaths as a consequence of economical misery.

The WTO system and its GATS principles represent another threat, whose serious consequences are already visible in the social and health sectors. These principles are now under implementation in the European Union via the new constitution and the Bolkestein Directive, whether slightly modified or not, releasing serious threats towards the quality of the social and health care systems.

Allyson Pollock (16) in UK has shown that even in affluent capitalist countries public services can face deterioration as a consequence of privatization. This is already obvious for the hospital sector in UK, where international companies enter to use the publicly accumulated fortunes for short term profits.

Conclusion

I hope this presentation has made clear the central role of democratically working trade unions in preventing illness, diseases and injuries on the one hand and promoting health and safety and an actively functioning democracy on the other.

If this continuous force is weakened or even eliminated, as we have seen in the US and UK and perhaps most strikingly in several low-income countries, the neoliberal horrors can propagate unhindered. In these years we have, i.e., in the Nordic countries, witnessed a considerable drift to the political right among the so-called workers' parties (Labour parties).

As a consequence of the 9-11 events in the US, whoever may have caused it, new laws with considerable limitations in fundamental democratic and civil rights have been passed in US as well as in the EU countries. Civil disobedience, demonstrations, strikes etc. can now easily be deemed expressions of terrorism and heavily punished.

All these types of so called "development" are fundamental threats to a flourishing future for humanity. I have to finish my presentation by, as strongly as possible, appealing to all workers and labor unions and their allies to resist these tendencies and acknowledge their historical responsibility to be the safeguard for human rights, health and safety included, and the vanguard for a brighter future, where capitalism is defeated and the working class comes to power.

REFERENCES:

1. Berkman, L. F., and Kawachi, I. Social Epidemiology. Oxford University Press, Oxford, 2000.
2. Breilh J. Epidemiología Critica. Ciencia emancipadora e interculturalidad. uenos Aires 2003: Lugar Editorial.
3. Elling, R. H. The Struggle for Workers' Health. Baywood, Amityville, N.Y.,1986.
4. Malerrapporten, Århus [The Painter Report, Aarhus], 1971, and Maler-rapport, København [The Painter Report, Copenhagen], 1972. In Danish.
5. Johansson, M., and Olsen, J. Helbredsforhold hos lakarbejdere i Snedker-&

Tømrerforbundets Århusafdeling [Health conditions of acid-curing enamel workers in the Aarhus branch of the Carpenters' and Woodworkers' Union]. Ugeskrift Laeger 137:916–918, 1975. In Danish.

6. Arlien-Søborg, P. Kronisk Toxisk Encefalopati hos bygningsmalere [Chronic Toxic Encephalopathy in Building Painters (summary and tables in English)]. Dissertation, Copenhagen, 1983.

7. Christiansen, J. M., et al. Opløsningsmidler i malerfaget [Organic Solvents in Housepainting Work: Health Damage among House Painters (English summary)]. Research report. Copenhagen, 1983.

8. Errebo-Knudsen, E. O., and Olsen, F. Organiske opløsningsmidler og præsenil demens (malersyndromet) [Organic Solvents and Pre-senile Dementia (Painter Syndrome)]. Joint representation of the oil industry. Copenhagen, 1984. In Danish.

9. Arbejdsmiljøgruppen, Rapport nr 2: Arbejdsmiljøundersøgelsen [The Working Environment Group, Report No. 2: The Working Environment Study], p. 28. Copenhagen, 1972. In Danish.

10. The Research Council of LO. Fagbevægelsen og forskningen [The Labor Movement and Research]. Copenhagen, 1975. In Danish.

11. Rossi, Ernest L.: "The Psychobiology of Gene Expression". WW Norton & Co., NY & London 2002

12. Farmer, Paul: "Pathologies of Power".University of California Press, 2003

13. Bulhan, Hussein Abdilahi: "Franz Fanon and the Psychology of Oppression". Plenum Press, NY & London 1985

14. Buchanan, David R.: "An Ethic for Health Promotion. Rethinking the sources of human wellbeing". Oxford University Press, NY & Oxford, 2000

15. "Understanding social inequalities in health". Marmot, M.G. 2003. Perspect.Biol.Med. vol. 46 3 suppl. s9-23

16. Pollock, Allyson M.: "NHS plc. The privatisation of our Health Care". Verso, London & NY 2004

Markets versus mental health: A case study of the inappropriateness of the mainstream health reform agenda

John Lister

The contradiction between the scale of the unmet need and the level and development of policy debate is especially stark in the case of mental health – quite possibly because of the close correlation between mental health and poverty on the one hand, and the social stigma widely attached to mental health patients on the other (Knapp et al 2002, Sturm and Gresenz 2002, Patel 2001, Weich and Lewis 1998, WHO 1996, WHO 1999, Brundtland 1999).

As a result, while mental health problems blight the lives of tens of millions of people around the world, policies for the development of mental health services appear to rate low on the list of priorities of health care reformers, even where they are included on the list at all.

Nor is the failure to address issues of mental health care restricted to the poorest countries. The contrast in attitude among the world's wealthier nations to the issues of mental health and those relating to ageing was summed up in the launch in 2001 of a 3-year Health Project by the OECD. This announced the intention to confront the growing challenges facing health policy and health care systems, and set out to measure and analyse the performance of health care systems in member countries. But while the project designated long-term care for frail elderly persons as a specific area of study, it made no reference at all to mental health, despite the fact that it is a substantial health issue among older people (OECD 2001).

Mental health care in wealthy countries

The problems and contradictions faced by capitalist societies in dealing with mental health reflect the fact that the inverse relationship between level of illness and ability to pay for treatment is as wide if not wider in mental health than any other area of care. The link between mental illness and poverty is well established, while it has been estimated in various contexts that between 10-30% of psychiatric service users with severe needs utilise as much as 80% of the services available (Torrey 1997; Lien 2003). These are also the people least likely to have well-paid formal sector jobs or the means to be covered by insurance, or able to pay fees to cover the sometimes extremely high costs of their care, which may be required for many years.

This means that the greater their level of health need, the less attractive a mental illness sufferer is as a client to a for-profit private sector provider, and the less easily such needs can be met within a market-style health care system or "managed care" (Chisholm and Stewart 1998). There are also indications that poverty and unemployment can serve to prolong the duration of mental illness, resulting in even higher costs of care (Weich and Lewis 1998).

The focus for policy makers and service providers therefore tends to switch away from those with the greatest needs to those with the least, or most manageable problems, and those already within the system. As one senior executive of a for-profit mental health service provider in the US summed up:

"You don't go looking for people who are going to be the highest risk unless you want to go bankrupt" (Quoted in Torrey 1997:125)

In 1990 Lave and Goldman noted that less than 3% of Medicare spending in the USA was on mental health, and that:

"policies regarding mental disorders differ from those for physical disorders. Coverage of mental disorders is more limited, and payment rules sometimes differ for specialty mental health providers" (Lave and Goldman 1990:20).

More recent studies confirm the ongoing pattern of unequal US health spending:

"mental health benefits in private health insurance plans are typically much less generous than benefits for physical health care services, with separate deductibles, higher coinsurance requirements, and lower annual and lifetime maxima" (Zuvekas et al 1998).

This approach appears to have largely continued among most of the key makers of health policy during the 1990s. In the more prosperous countries, where the possibility of using new, improved but more expensive drugs as part of a new system of community-based care could be financially feasible, there has been a reluctance to channel the necessary resources into mental health: attention and investment has tended to remain more focused on acute surgical and medical treatment.

Modern psychiatry, which developed in the post-war period with the growing use of new drugs, notably Chlorpromazine, in the 1950s, has been one of the first to embrace the notion of "evidence-based" practice, running randomised controlled trials which established the effectiveness of anti-depressants and anti-psychotic drugs in the 1960s (Rivett 1998, Geddes et al 1997). The growing effectiveness of the drugs, especially the more modern anti-psychotic drugs with fewer harmful side-effects, made it possible to devise new, community-based services to replace much of the institutionalised care in large psychiatric hospitals1 (WHO 1999). The new generation of anti-depressants are substantially more costly – but also claimed to be more efficacious than the previous type of drugs they replace: control of costs needs to be seen in a wider rather than a narrower sense if patients are to benefit and long-term costs are to be contained (Stewart 1998).

However the driving force in mental health care reforms is not technique and innovation, but the quest to minimise spending: no matter how eager the pharmaceutical corporations may be to capitalise on their investment, new drugs that cost more will only be used when it is shown they can generate savings for those holding the purse strings. Even within the relatively neglected area of mental health, the care of older people is even less of a priority in the allocation of resources. In the UK, research into Alzheimer's disease receives just £11 per Alzheimer's patient, compared with the £289 per cancer patient (Salari 2003).

In Britain, government policy since 1959 has looked to develop "community care" as the model for mental health – a policy reinforced by then Health Minister Enoch Powell in a landmark speech in 1961, in which he proclaimed the old-style Victorian "asylums" to be the "defences we have to storm" if a new model of care was to emerge (Ham 1999, Caldwell et al 1998). In practice the lead in closing down the large mental hospitals was given by the Italian government, beginning in the 1970s (Knapp et al 2002). More than 40 years later, however, it is not only the British government that has lagged behind in implementing its own self-proclaimed policies.

A "backwater" specialty

Over the same period psychiatric medicine has failed to attain the public prestige and professional predominance that has been accorded to other medical specialties, despite the high hopes expressed in a *Lancet* editorial back in 1963, which proclaimed that:

> "From being a backwater, ignored as much by the rest of medicine as by the public at large, psychiatry is becoming one of the major specialties" (cited in Rivett 1998:159).

There is little doubt that one of the reasons for the almost universally low status of psychiatry and mental health compared with other sectors of health care (notably the prestigious specialties such as cardiac surgery, orthopaedics and other acute hospital treatment) is linked to the generally low economic status and often the low social status or social exclusion of mental illness sufferers.

There are very few wealthy patients who can realistically be expected to pay the full costs for their own mental health care: any expansion or enhancement of service provision therefore requires either an increase in overall premium payments by those in private insurance schemes, or increased state spending, whether funded from social insurance or general taxation.

Even in the US, which has the most private of health care systems, public spending covered 53% of all mental health treatment costs in 1996, while private insurance covered only around a quarter (Hogan 1999). Torrey (1997) estimates that the public share of US mental health spending is even higher.

In Britain, the closure of the asylums was also urged on by mental health campaigners concerned at growing evidence that long-term incarceration in a large-scale institution could deprive patients of any chance of regaining a normal life (Caldwell et al 1998, Lister 1999). But while the closures appeared to unite the Thatcher government with the liberal and libertarian campaigners, the vital issue of resources for new community-based services was overlooked.

During the 1980s, when the programme of "downsizing" and closure of the large mental hospitals began in earnest (40% of psychiatric beds closed 1982-92) it was at first assumed that a community-based service could be as cheap or even cheaper than hospital beds.

This approach was harshly criticised in 1985 by an all-party committee of MPs, who insisted that:

"A decent community-based service for mentally ill ... people cannot be provided at the same overall cost as the present services. ...

"Community care on the cheap would prove worse in many respects than the pattern of services to date" (Commons Social Services Committee 1985, xiv).

Any change in the configuration of mental health services required investment – in new drugs, in the training of staff to work in new community-based services, and in housing and alternative accommodation for people who would otherwise have been long-stay hospital in-patients.

US shrinks its mental health services

A very similar set of problems seem to have also arisen in the USA, where the market and its associated ideology have reigned supreme. Torrey (1997:8-9) shows the extraordinary and rapid "deinstitutionalisation" which reduced the number of in-patients in psychiatric beds from 558,239 in 1955 to just 71,619 in 1994 – over a period in which the total US population increased by 50 percent.

Not only were the psychiatric institutions emptied, they were also closed down, leaving no services for later patients who would previously have been admitted. Even allowing for 10,000 in-patients in Community Mental Health Centres, and another 40,000 in psychiatric beds in general hospitals, Torrey argues that more than three quarters of a million severely mentally ill people – "more than the population of San Francisco" – are now living in the community who would have been hospitalised 40 years ago (Torrey 1997:9).

Perhaps equally concerning is the fact that in the world's largest and leading developed economy, according to the US National Advisory Mental Health Council, only around 60% of severely mentally ill adults – suffering from conditions including schizophrenia – received treatment in any given year.

This means around 2.2 million people with severe mental illness receiving no treatment (cited by Torrey 1997:6). The problem is also compounded by the fact that as Ustun (2000) argues, nearly half of those who need mental health treatment do not seek it, while many of those who do suffer from the side-effects of the cheapest available medicines, social stigma, poor continuity of care, and inadequate follow-up from under-resourced community teams.

One conspicuous area of underinvestment, the impact of wide-scale drug abuse, and its knock-on effects on law and order in the USA, has frequently been discussed in the mass media. Cartwright estimates the total cost of this to US society at $110 billion in 1995. However spending on drug abuse treatment amounted to just 1% of health insurance costs (Cartwright 1999).

Far from addressing or resolving the gaps and problems in mental health services, government policy and the emergence of "managed care" and for-profit medicine have simply made things worse in the USA. The introduction of Medicaid in 1965 with a provision to fund mental health care was seized upon by states as a way to shift cost burdens onto the federal government.

Whereas in 1963 98% of mental illness treatment was funded by state and local governments, Torrey argues that by 1994 the federal government was underwriting 62% of the total costs, largely through Medicare and Medicaid. This served to speed up the inappropriate discharge of tens of thousands of patients from hospital care; fuelled the expansion of low quality and institutional nursing home care; encouraged the expansion of psychiatric beds in general hospitals – which can be substantially more expensive than publicly-run psychiatric hospitals; and led to a disjointed system:

> "The result is the most expensive, yet least coordinated system of psychiatric services in the Western world" (Torrey 1997:105)

By 1995, the US mental health managed care industry was described by the *Wall Street Journal* as a $2 billion industry with potential for additional growth, "boasting margins of 15% and more".

In part this profitability has been created by "skimming" to take in only the least ill patients, and "dumping" those seen as higher risks (Torrey 1997).

Markets and mental health

The market-style reforms in Britain and in many countries during the 1990s have raised a different, though related series of questions: can such a system result in a progressive reform of mental health services? Hadley and Goldman (1995) appear to answer this in the negative.

These Pennsylvania University researchers were among the first to question the impact of market-style reforms on mental health care in Britain, finding that the situation of perverse incentives and multiple payers had created a "difficult and complex" system from a relatively simple one, and left clinicians struggling to provide services:

> "The situation is therefore reminiscent of the mental
> health system in the United States, where funding and
> responsibilities have been fragmented and the relation
> between specialist services and primary health care has
> become poorly defined and in many cases non-existent"
> (Hadley and Goldman 1995).

More recently Lien (2003) has explored the effects of market-style policies on mental health services in Norway. He notes that these reforms strong focus on increasing the productivity of the acute hospital sector.

However mental health was specifically exempted from Norway's new payment-by-results funding system, making it less likely that – in merged healthcare trusts spanning both general medicine and mental health – any expansion of mental health services would be seen as a financially attractive prospect by providers.

Lien argues that mental health, as an area of health care in which the level of risk is especially hard to predict, is in general especially unsuited to conventional market forces. It was excluded from the system of prospective payment based on diagnostic related groups when this was introduced in the USA.

In New Zealand and Australia there is evidence that payment by diagnostic related group tends to lead to misclassification of patients, to make it seem as if their condition is more serious and complex – and thus qualify for higher payments.

Lien also notes that the introduction of new funding mechanisms in the USA through Medicare in the 1980s served to reduce average length of stay in psychiatric hospitals, but also led to a rising rate of readmission.

The transition to outpatient and day case treatment of patients who would previously have been admitted to hospital can cause problems for others: while it may be cheaper as far as service providers are concerned, some of these savings come at the expense of unpaid carers who support patients between episodes of treatment. Only in the longer term – if at all – do these carers see the benefit of their increased effort (Creed et al 1997).

However Trieman and colleagues have shown properly planned and resourced care in the community can be beneficial for most patients and has few detrimental effects on their new neighbours (Trieman et al 1999).

Murray and colleagues, assessing a community team's work warn that many of those most needing treatment do not seek it, even from community teams in England:

"Our single most important shortcoming has been the failure systematically to reassess patients who may not seek help" (Murray et al 1996).

Mental health care is perhaps the most extreme example of the need to invert the traditional hierarchy of professional-led services, to empower the service users, and enlist their active participation and cooperation, both to sustain their own treatment and to help shape the services they require (Gureje and Alem 2000). Yet this runs so far counter to the existing power relations within the health care systems that progress on these issues has at best been slow and uneven (Simpson and House 2002, Lund and Flisher 2001, WHR 2001). Health reformers have in general not even begun to address this issue.

Mental health in developing countries

If discussed at all in the context of developing countries, mental health care has been largely dealt with as an adjunct to the more central issue of establishing a minimum package of primary health care services, and setting up new structures of user fees as a device to establish various forms of health insurance.

Perhaps because it doesn't easily fit into any market-style reform package, mental health has also remained largely neglected as a subject for policy research by the otherwise active global agencies and consultancies. A search of the World Bank's 14,000 on-line publications for the term "mental health" early in 2003 drew just 19 references, none dealing in any depth with policy issues.

The extensive final collected works of the USAID-funded Partnerships for Health Reform also contain only a few scant references to mental health or psychiatric services. PHR publications in general make only occasional and passing references to mental health care: a report of a Social Health Insurance Working Group, meeting in Zimbabwe in 1998, for example, examines the possible outlines of a benefits package to be secured through SHI, but asks (without attempting to answer the question):

"Should mental health services be included?" (Kress et al 1998:32).

Another PHR study notes without further comment that private sector health insurance policies "generally exclude dental and mental health coverage…" The same authors point out that private policies also exclude treatment for other conditions which are commonly assigned to the care of mental health services – alcoholism, Alzheimer's and bulimia (Hollander and Rauch 1998:15).

A similar picture of exclusion also emerges from the privatised insurance system which the post-Sandinista government in Nicaragua introduced in 1994, to cover just 6% of the population (Bitran et al 2000). Cohen contrasts the radical and progressive changes that were ushered in to Nicaragua's mental health care under the Sandinista government, which achieved a drastic reduction in the "custodial" treatment of psychiatric patients, with the subsequent reversal of policy after the right wing regained power in 1990:

"Mental health services were eliminated from primary care. Psychiatric patients cannot be admitted to general hospitals, and conditions in the national mental health hospital have deteriorated because of severe budget cuts" (Cohen 2001:19).

Mental health on the periphery

The peripheral importance of mental health to pro-market reformers of health services is again underlined when a PHR-funded study on Rwanda mentions in passing that the country has three public referral hospitals and "one mental health care hospital": its subsequent policy analysis does not discuss the integration of that hospital or mental health care into the pre-payment system that is the main focus of the study (Schneider et al 2000).

Another PHR report on Rwanda details the imposition of a $15 fee for each electroencephalogram, and a sliding scale of fees (ranging from $1.50 to $9) for consultations at the country's first mental health outpatient centre. The report fails to make any comparison between these charges and the average income of Rwandans in greatest need of mental health care – but nevertheless concludes by asserting that:

"Patients are willing to pay a fee for services they perceive as valuable" (PHR 2000c).

The fact that psychotropic drugs are available at a subsidised price from the clinic, whereas they are far more expensive if purchased through private pharmacies, is not recognised by the authors as the decisive factor in this 'willingness to pay'. The exception that underlines the general rule of the marginalisation of mental health care within the debates on health sector reform is a PHR study of Jamaica. It makes the point that the authors deliberately set out to include mental health services in their survey of the impact of policies on the "indigent" because:

"There is a dearth of data on this chronic illness in Jamaica. Mental illness is also proving to be very costly to the Jamaican government since it incurs the longest average hospitalisation for chronic illness" (Henry-Lee and Yearwood 1999:xiii).

The authors report that schizophrenia and delusional disorders accounted for over 9% of inpatient care, with an average length of stay of almost 92 days. They note that France singles out mental health for exemption from relatively high co-payments which apply to other sectors of health care, and point out that a number of countries in practice also recognise the difficulty in charging mental health patients the high costs of continuing care and of in-patient treatment. And they endorse the view that for as long as mental health consisted largely of "custodial" in-patient treatment it had no place in health insurance.

Warning that the Jamaican government's National Health Insurance Plan is seriously under-funded to deal with the numbers of people suffering chronic conditions, the authors also warn of the detrimental effects that are likely to arise from government plans to halve the number of in-patients in the country's main psychiatric hospital, unless adequate services are put in place to support those who would be sent home (Henry-Lee and Yearwood 1999:35).

It is hard to avoid the conclusion from the approach in each of the above studies that mental health is in general seen as a side-issue or an optional extra by governments and by many of the key global players in health policy reform.

A world wide problem

In the late 1990s the WHO, the one global agency that has given a high profile to mental health issues, began to draw attention to the size of the gap that was opening up in provision for this area of health care, especially in the developing countries. The WHO summed up the situation in 2001:

"Globally, the mental health resources in countries present a dismal picture of severe shortage and neglect. Often the services and resources are one tenth to one hundredth of what is needed" (WHO 2001d:4).

The most recent available WHO figures show that mental health disorders account for 12% of all disability-adjusted life years and almost a third of the years lived with a disability. They account for six of the top 20 causes of disease burden among the world's population aged 15-44 (Knapp et al 2003) and for five of the ten leading causes of disability world wide (manic depression, schizophrenia, bipolar disorders, alcohol use, obsessive compulsive disorders) (WHO 1999).

At any one time as many as 1.5 billion people world-wide are suffering from mental or neurological disorders, or from problems related to alcohol and drug abuse. It is estimated that as many as one on four people on the globe will suffer such a disorder at some point in their lives (WHO 1996b). There is also a link to ageing, with the WHO warning that the increase in life-expectancy brings with it greater risk of age-related mental illnesses (WHO 1996g).

Numbers suffering from senile dementia in Africa, Asia and Latin America are projected to increase from 20 million in 1990 to at least 80 million by 2025. Urbanisation, which intensifies rates of abuse of alcohol and illicit drugs, and leaves tens of millions of adults and children homeless in sprawling "megacities": it also erodes traditional forms of family and social support for elderly people and those with mental illness (WHO 1996c).

Again the inverse care law

Once again the available information – in this case much of it painstakingly collated by the WHO, which has compiled a comparative study covering 185 of its 191 member states – underlines the prevalence of the "inverse care law", both at national level and internationally. At the root of much mental illness is the constant pressure of grinding poverty: as Brundtland (1999) argues "For the WHO, mental well being is an integral part of mental health," and poverty is a major obstacle to such well-being.

Worse: the chances of having to pay "out of pocket" for any mental health services are the greatest for people living in the poorest countries. Cash payment without the benefit of any insurance or public funding was the most common means of financing care in 40% of low income countries, compared with 12% in lower middle income, zero in higher middle and just 2.9% of high income countries.

The problem is worst in Africa and South East Asia (WHO Atlas 2001). While the median number of psychiatrists available in all countries is one per 100,000 population, the high income countries actually have NINE per 100,000, while the poorest African Region countries average just one psychiatrist per two million people. 44% of the world's population has access to less than one psychiatric nurse per 100,000 people[2] (WHO 2001).

All of the 18 countries which reported in excess of 10 psychiatric hospital beds per 10,000 population were either OECD countries or in Europe. By far the highest use of in-patient beds was recorded by Japan (28.4 beds per 10,000 population) and Belgium (25), while the next heaviest user of hospital care was Canada on 19.3. By contrast the average bed availability for the whole of Africa was 0.78 per 10,000 population, and even this is distorted by the atypical and relatively high bed numbers in Mauritius (8) and South Africa (4.5).

South Africa topped the African provision for psychiatric nursing staff, with 7.5 nurses per 100,000 population, but many African countries had fewer than one per 100,000. 24 wealthier countries reported coverage three times or more higher than Africa's best, with a highest level in Finland (176) followed by the UK (104) Netherlands (99) and Ireland (96.5).

The inequality reaches beyond the issue of beds and staff: a third of the world's population has no access to essential drugs for treating mental health problems, including psychotropic drugs. The problem is even worse in the rural areas of the poorest countries.

In India only 20% of people suffering from schizophrenia and epilepsy received treatment, compared with an average of 80% in the established market economies. But mental health remains the poor relation of health services: only an estimated 35% of patients suffering from depression receive treatment, even in countries with well-developed health care systems (WHO 1999b).

WHO researchers found that 40% of countries had no explicit mental health policy at all, and a third had no mental health programme. 38% provided no community-based mental health care, while 33% did not report having a specific mental health budget, and a similar percentage allocate less than one percent of health spending to mental health: most devoted less than five percent (WHO World Health Report 2001).

The user fees which are being promoted as the solution to funding problems in other parts of the health care system are central to the continued exclusion of millions of mental illness sufferers from the care they require. Even more than the frail elderly, it is those with mental illness who find themselves outside the health care framework, looking in, while the attention of reformers is firmly focused elsewhere, on issues affecting acute hospitals, insurance systems and the role of private sector providers.

1 Torrey (1997) argues that the biggest impact on deinstitutionalisation of care in the USA came not from new drugs but from changes in federal funding of mental health and the opportunity for widespread "cost shifting" by states.
2 The WHO's 2001 survey of mental health care provision around the world underlines the stark inequalities that prevail between the poorest and richest countries.

References

Bitran y Asociados (Ubilla G, Espinosa C and Bitran R) (2000) 'The use of capitation payment by the Social Security Institute and previsional medical enterprises in Nicaragua', Major Applied Research 2, Working Paper 3 PHR, Abt Associates, Bethesda Ma

Brundtland GH, 1999, Raising awareness, fighting stigma, improving care: Brundtland unveils new WHO global strategies for mental health, Press Release WHO Geneva, Nov 12 1998

Caldwell K, Francome C and Lister J (1998) *The Envy of the World.* NHS Support Federation, London

Cartwright WS, 1999, Book Review: Methods for the Economic Evaluation of health care programmes, Drummond MF et al, *Journal of Mental Health Policy and Economics*, 2: 43

Chisholm A and Ford R (2004) *Transforming mental health care.* Sainsbury Centre for Mental Health, London

Cohen A, 2001, *The effectiveness of mental health services in primary care: the view from the developing world*, Nations for Mental Health, WHO, Geneva

Commons Social Services Committee, 1985, Session 1984-85 *Community Care*, Vol 1, London HMSO

Creed F, Mbaya P, Lancashire S, Tomenson B, Williams B, Holme S, 1997, Cost effectiveness of day and inpatient psychiatric treatment: results of a randomised controlled trial, *BMJ*, 314: 1381 (May 10)

Doyal L, 1979, *The Political Economy of Health*, Pluto Press, London

Drache D, Sullivan T , 1999, *Health Reform Public success, private failure*, Routledge, London

Dyer G, 2003a, AstraZeneca linked to US healthcare scheme fraud, *Financial Times*, January 31

Dyer G, 2003c, AstraZeneca pays $355m in sales fraud probe, *Financial Times*, June 21-22

Geddes J, Reynolds S, Streiner D, Szatmari P, 1997, Evidence based practice in mental health, *BMJ*, 315: 1483-1484 (December 6)

Gureje O, Alem A, 2000, Mental health policy development in Africa, *Bull WHO*, 78; 4: 475-482

Hadley TR, Goldman H, 1995, Effect of recent health and social service policy reforms on Britain's mental health system, *BMJ*, 311: 1556-1558, December 9

Ham C (1999) *Health Policy in Britain.* (4th edition) Macmillan, London

Henry-Lee A, Yearwood A, 1999, Protecting the poor and the medically indigent under health insurance: a case study of Jamaica, Small Applied Research No.6, PHR, Abt Associates, Bethesda Ma

Hogan MF, 1999, Public sector mental health care: new challenges, *Health Affairs*, Vol 18; 5: 106-111

Hollander N, Rauch M, 1998, Assessment of third party payers in Jordan, Technical Report No.27, PHR, Abt Associates, Bethesda Ma

Ireland D, 2003, The bad doctor: Bill Frist's long record of corporate vice, *LA\Weekly*, January 10-16 www.laweekly.com/accessed 12.7.03

Knapp M, 2002, Mental health: familiar challenges, unprecedented opportunities?, *eurohealth*, 8:1 21-24 (Winter 2001-2002)

Knapp M, McDaid D, Mossialos E, Thornicroft G, 2003, *Mental health policy and practice across Europe: the future direction of Mental Health Care, Proposal for analytical study*, WHO European Observatory on Health Care Systems www.who.dk/eprise/main/WHO/Progs/OBS/Studies/200211.htm, (23.02.03)

Kress DH, Fairbank A, Atim C, 1998, Social Health Insurance Working Group, Meeting in Zimbabwe January 28-30 1998, PHR Workshop Report No.1, PHR, Abt Associates, Bethesda, Ma

Lave JR, Goldman HH, 1990, Medicare Financing for Mental Health Care, *Health Affairs*, Spring 1990

Lien L, 2003, Financial and organisational reforms in the health sector: implications for the financing and management of mental health care services, *Health Policy*, Vol 63(1) 73-80, January

Lister J (1999) *Mental Health in London: The Care Gap*. UNISON, London May 27

Lund C, Flisher AJ, 2001, South African mental health process indicators, *Journal of Mental Health Policy and Economics*, 4; 1: 9-16

Murray V, Walker HW, Mitchell C, Pelosi AJ, 1996, Needs for care from a demand led community psychiatric service: a study of patients with major mental illness, *BMJ*, 312: 1582-1586, June 22

OECD, 2001 (b), OECD Health Project, OECD Paris, May 2001

Palast G, 1999, Sickness at the heart of private medicine, *The Observer Business*, April 25: 10

Patel D, 2004, Who's going to heal Ngilu's ailing Ministry of Health? *East African Standard*, Thursday October 7, www.eastandard.net/archives, accessed 27.03.05

PHR, 2000, Health Insurance models becoming more popular in Africa, *Healthwatch* (Abt Associates newsletter), Fall 2000

Rivett G (1998) *From Cradle to Grave*. Kings Fund, London

Salari N, 2003a, Are health and care services ready for a surge in Alzheimer's cases? *Community Care*, 16-17, 28 August-3Sept

Schneider P, Diop FP, Bucyana S, 2000, Development and implementation of pre-payment schemes in Rwanda, Technical Report No. 45, PHR, Abt Associates, Bethesda Ma

Simpson EL, House AO, 2002, Involving users in the delivery and evaluation of mental health services: a systematic review, *BMJ*, 325: 1265 (November 30)

Stewart A, 1998, Cost effectiveness of SSRIs: a European perspective, *Journal of*

Mental Health Policy and Economics, 1: 41-49

Sturm R, Gresenz CR, 2002, Relations of income inequality and family income to chronic medical conditions and mental health disorders: national survey, *BMJ*, 324: 1-5, (January 5)

Torrey EF, 1997, *Out of the shadows: confronting America's mental illness crisis*, John Wiley, New York

Trieman N, Leff J, Glover G, 1999, Outcome of long stay psychiatric patients resettled in the community: prospective cohort study, *BMJ*, 319: 13-16, July 3

US Department of Justice, 2003, Largest health care fraud case in U.S. history settled: HCA investigation nets record total of $1.7 billion, *Press Release*, June 26 www.usdoj.gov, accessed 4.05.05

Ustun TB, 2000, Mainstreaming mental health, *Bull WHO*, 78; 4: 412

Valkin V, Bowe C, 2003, Reputation of US business is tarnished again, *Financial Times*, June 13

Weich S, Lewis G, 1998, Poverty, unemployment and common mental disorders: population based cohort study, *BMJ*, 317:115-9 (July 11)

WHO, 1996b, *Mental Health, Fact Sheet No. 130*, WHO Geneva August

WHO, 1996c, *Mental health and demographic factors, Fact Sheet No. 131*, WHO Geneva August

WHO, 1996g, *Psychiatry of the Elderly: a consensus statement*, WHOMNH/MND/96.7 Geneva, February

WHO, 1999 d, *The 'newly defined' burden of mental problems, Fact Sheet No 217*, WHO Geneva April

WHO, 1999b , Raising awareness, fighting stigma, improving care, *Press Release*, November 12, WHO Geneva

WHO, 2000, *World Health Report*

WHO , 2001, *Atlas: country profiles on mental health resources 2001*, WHO Geneva

WHO, 2001 d, *Project Atlas: Mapping mental health services around the world*, Fact Sheet, WHO Geneva

Zuvekas SH, Banthin JS, Selden TM, 1998, Mental health parity: what are the gaps in coverage?, *Journal of Mental Health Policy and Economics*, 1: 135-146

Health Care in Croatia – Market or social values?

Aleksandar Dzakula, MD, Luka Voncina, MSc, MD, Professor
Jadranka Mustajbegovic, PhD, MD, Nikolina Radakovic, MD

ABSTRACT:

In the 1980s, self-government was developed as a special
management form for the health care system. The system of
self-governing was based on direct citizens' participation in
decision making and regional decentralization. Political
reforms related to the onset of transition in Croatia in 1990,
and the struggle for independence gained in 1991, led to
reforms of the overall system, including health care. One of
the measures introduced was the centralization of health
care, justified by the lack of co-operation and control as
well as severe financial difficulties. This period was distin-
guished by an orientation towards war-related health issues
and target groups. A new stage in health care reforms was
undertaken in 1993: this organised health insurance as
national system, defined (national, and regional) ownership
in health care and introduced privatisation. The central
administration kept very tight control over health care
through finances and by-laws, but the main idea was to
introduce market principles into the health care system.
However the economic crisis 1995-2000 again emphasised
social issues and political dimension of health care. In 2002,
national complementary insurance was introduced to cover
co-payments, and many vulnerable groups were given free

access to care, even complementary insurance. This change was recognized as patient friendly, but caused a rapid increase of the health care expenditures. Therefore the most recently announced reforms stress the need to cut costs, introduce higher participation fees and more market values in health care. Croatia has a heath care system that recognized many social issues and vulnerable groups. The long lasting financial crisis, along with a partially reformed system and constant increase in health care expenditures face decision makers every few years with need to make changes in health policy.

1.0 CROATIA BETWEEN SOCIALISM AND MARKET ECONOMY

1.1. Self Government

Before the beginning of the 1990s Croatian society was based on socialist values, with workers-employees playing the most prominent role in ensuring social progress.(1) Workers were the most active part of the population and were present in almost all aspects of public life. In the sector of public services it was impossible to assess many fields of social life according to market laws or comparison of results achieved. The need for such assessment was recognized, and the Constitution defined the category of free exchange of labour as a new social relation. In order to establish and carry out free exchange of labour, self-governing communities of interest were founded for separate fields of general social importance. Those communities were active in the following fields: education, science, culture, health care, social welfare, pension and disability insurance, residence, utilities and economic infrastructure.

The model of self-government was first introduced in health care by the Health Insurance Act (1974), and was fully governed by the unified Health Care and Health Insurance Act (1980). Self-managing Communities of interest were established by contracting between users (employees and citizens) and health care providers. They were aimed at organizing and financing the health system, including health insurance. Community Assemblies comprised representatives of users, providers and local authorities. They were responsible for key issues in the health care system of the area the community was founded for and its decision-making policy was based on consensus.

The model of Self- management (Fig. 1) in health care was specific in two ways:

● It operated a model of joint decision-making policy by both users and providers.

● Communities were run by their Assemblies that comprised representatives of users and health care providers.

Planning, management and financing (of health insurance) were consolidated. Communities of interest took over the central role in organizing and financing health care. Such a consolidated model of decision-making and financing was also operative on the national level, governed by the unified Health Care and Health Insurance Act (1980).

Service users, through their representatives, had direct influence in deciding about health care, enabling them to play a more successful role in meeting their requirements. User participation in decision-making was a unique model that activated the community in health care. Self-government in health was a peculiar model and as such served as a topic for many analyses and discussions. On the one hand, advantages of the system were emphasized: equity and user participation in decision-making, responsiveness to specific local requirements. On the other hand, financial difficulties, inequalities in the country's regions and inadequate distribution of resources were pointed out as drawbacks. (2)

Fig. 1. Organisational structure of the Self-governing communities

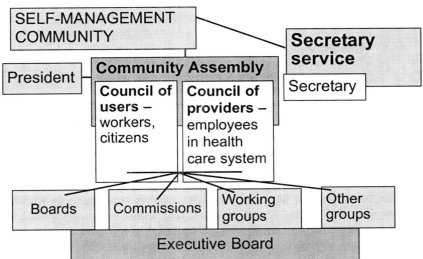

Source: Letica S. *Health policy during a crisis*. Naprijed, Zagreb 1989, p.208

1.2. Transition and Centralisation

Self- management was based on the following principles:
- Public ownership of self- management health providers
- Focusing on primary care
- Continuous development and expansion of health care, "moral of progress".

However, for many reasons, development and expansion of the health system did not go as planned, but were checked by financial and professional crisis and lack of management accountability. Debts in the health care system rose to US$ 180 million by 1990 and such tendencies could in no way relate to the "moral of progress" – the third principle of self-government. Organizational analysis showed some weak points of the implemented decentralized model. These were primarily:
- Deficit of funds and financial crisis of the system
- Inequality in regions
- Inadequate distribution of resources. (3)

The inherited decentralized health system organized in local communities and based on labour associations was bound to change. In the year 1990, decentralized authorities of local communities (self-governing health communities of interest) were transferred to the national level and the newly founded Croatian Republic Fund of Health Insurance and Health Care. The Fund was based on the former Association of Self-governing Communities of Interest, which was responsible for control and joint interests of local communities on the national level. The reform transferred decision-making from local authorities to the central national authority. Furthermore, health financing was centralised and governed by the Republic Fund. (4)

1.3. The Aggression and War 1991-1995

During the war which followed national independence in 1991, Croatia suffered extensive humanitarian crisis (Table 1) and material damage. By mid-1995, over 16,000 Croatian citizens had been killed in the war and over 30,000 had been made permanent invalids. A survey in Croatia in March 1996 counted 361,774 displaced persons and refugees. Direct damage (excluding many indirect effects) was estimated by the State Commission for War Damage Inventory and Assessment to amount to US $27 billion. For example, nearly 10% of housing stock was destroyed or damaged as well as a considerable amount of public service infrastructure. (4)

After the deep crisis during the 1980s the period between 1988 and 1990, however, marked an upturn and introduction of market economy. According to official statistics, GDP per capita amounted to US $5,106, while the unemployment rate was 9.3%. Democratic changes and election of parliamentary power brought about additional freedom in economy. Nevertheless, growing political crisis and upsurge of war made economic recovery impossible. Massive destruction during the war and the inadequate privatisation model of state ownership and companies had an extremely negative effect on Croatian economy.

The political system and the war enabled politics to influence major economic decisions. Poorly implemented privatization and unattractive political decisions resulted in Croatia's political and economic lagging behind neighbouring countries in the 90s. The fall in GDP, steady growth of unemployment, closing down work places and unbearable public expenditure indicate how severe the recession was. (5)

Soaring unemployment and number of the retired due to early retirement led to an extremely unfavourable ratio of the employed contributing to the state funds, compared to those receiving from them. In 1999 the number of people entitled to retirement allowance rose sharply to 989,000, while the number of the employed fell dramatically to 1,364,495. In such difficult economic conditions the state tried to preserve social peace by heavily burdening the budget to keep a large number of employees in state administration and public institutions.

Table 1. Inhabitants of the Republic of Croatia who do not generate income (1994)

Displaced persons	247,185
Refugees	272,383
Unemployed	245,634
Retirement beneficiaries	731,922
Social welfare beneficiaries	300,000
TOTAL	1,797124

(displaced + refugees)/population = 10.84 %

(persons non generating income)/employed=1.76

Those measures only aggravated the situation and deepened the recession: unemployment rose to over 20% and industrial production fell. (4)

1.4. Health Care Reform after 1993

Despite the deepening economic crisis and the war aggression on Croatia health care reform that started in 1993. The reform inherited most of the changes introduced in 1990, which were based on health trends from the 1980s. The 1990 reform established a new set of strategic relations in the health care system and passage of new legislation was needed to define further details and guidelines on reforms and foundations of the system.

The inherited system kept values of social equality, but had several drawbacks: lack of cost-effectiveness, control, and systematic quality control. Reforms were therefore aimed at creating a system with balanced market and social values in health care. This was to be achieved through privatisation and changes in public services – centralized decision-making and control and local resource management. (6) Such a system was believed to be elastic and dynamic enough to meet the requirements of the transition period.

For such a reformed system basic principles were defined: all-inclusiveness, continuity, and availability. Direct reforms were brought about by the Health Care Act and the Health Insurance Act in 1993.

2.0. CURRENT SITUATION: MARKET or SOCIAL JUSTICE?

2.1. Health Insurance

Croatia operates a Social Health Insurance system (elementary health insurance) that covers the major part of public expenditure for health care services, with a single publicly owned sickness fund – the Croatian Institute for Health Insurance (HZZO) for the entire population of the country. The total amount of funds allocated for health care (funded from elementary health insurance) is annually determined by the state budget and collected through the state treasury. The HZZO receives funds for elementary insurance from the state budget. Those funds originate from two main sources: payroll contributions (15% of gross salary, paid by all employees) and funds collected by general taxation.

According to the Croatian Ministry of Health and Social Affairs, salary contributions form more than 80% of the total of funds the state allocates to the elementary health insurance fund. (7) Therefore, while primarily based on the Bismarck model, the Croatian funding system displays characteristics specific to both Bismarck and Beveridge-like models, primarily due to the high number of individuals that do not financially contribute to the fund (retired, students, unemployed, etc.) through payroll contributions.

The 2002 health care law introduced voluntary Complementary Health Insurance into the funding system. Until 2004 this was legally offered exclusively by the HZZO: the premium for complementary insurance was (and currently still is) community rated and set at HRK 80 (cca EUR 11) per month, retired HRK 50 (cca EUR 7) per month. Complementary insurance restores full rights to free health care at the point of use in HZZO contracted providers. It can be paid by employers or employees and is fully tax deductible. HZZO collects premiums for complementary health insurance on its own through a separate account.

In 2003 Complementary health insurance was marketed solely by the HZZO and was purchased by 729,915 citizens, roughly 16 % of the Croatian population (8). Complementary health insurance – as could have been expected, because it was instituted as voluntary insurance with a community rate premium – pooled higher than average risks due to adverse selection (i.e. 51.65% of insured in 2003 were retired). Nevertheless, it created financial surpluses of HRK 144,000,000 (EUR 19,433,198) in 2002 and HRK 17,178,659 (EUR 2,272,309) in 2003 (8,9)

Although official data are currently not publicly available, government officials' statements indicate that in 2004 Complementary insurance accumulated a net financial deficit of HRK 137,000,000 (EUR 18,293,497) and that it has from 2004 on ceased being financially sustainable.

This is not surprising, taking into consideration the composition of its ensured population: already in 2003 it had attracted a disproportional amount of heavy spenders which had serious implications for its sustainability. Thus, it could be argued that Complementary health insurance is actually subsidized by the government, primarily as a measure of maintaining peace between the government and its social partners – trade unions, associations of patients, etc.

The 2005 amendments to the Health Insurance Law were heavily debated by various political parties and other organizations representing interested parties such as medical professionals and patients. They have further increased the co-payments schedule from 2002, by introducing "administrative fees" into the system of finance.

All patients, with the exception of children under 18 and the disabled (with invalidity over 80%), are required to pay deductibles of HRK 5 or HRK 10 (cca EUR 0.7 and EUR 1.4) (charged by their respective GP) for obtaining certain products and services, such as a prescription or a referral to a specialist. If a patient bypasses the gate keeping system by seeking care directly from a hospital emergency ward without prior consultation with his GP, then specialist consultations in emergency departments not judged to be of an emergency nature are also subject to an administrative fee of HRK 10 (cca EUR 1.4). The maximum amount of "administrative fees" that can be charged to a patient is HRK 30 (cca EUR 4) per month. Further referrals, prescriptions etc. are free of charge.

2.2. Private Sector

The inflow of private funds and user charges into the Croatian health care system originates from four sources:
- private health insurance,
- co-payments to providers contracted by HZZO,
- out of pocket payments to providers not contracted by HZZO
- and informal payments.

In 2002, the World Health Organization estimated private expenditure on health at 18.6% of total expenditure on health (10). According to the Croatian Ministry of Health and Social Affairs, private consumption in health care has remained at 2% of total GDP until 2005 (1). Patients are required to pay out of pocket to privately owned providers (not contracted by HZZO), and if they do not have complementary health insurance, co-payments to providers contracted by HZZO for services not fully covered or not covered by elementary health insurance. Although informal payments do not form a part of the official funding system and are furthermore illegal, published research (11) suggests that it would not be realistic to deny their existence in Croatia, as seems to be the case in the greater part of Central and Eastern Europe (12).

Private insurers collect premiums for supplementary insurance that can be used with contracted private or publicly owned providers. As in most European Union countries, private health insurance plays a marginal role in funding health care in Croatia. In 2002, private health insurers reported annual revenues of HRK 962 million (cca EUR 130 million) or roughly 6% of total health expenditure (13)

Prior to 2002, individuals with annual income over a certain limit (annually determined by the Minister of Health) were allowed to opt out from the compulsory health insurance system and to insure with privately owned insurers instead. The 2002 Health care law prohibited opt-out and confined the benefits of private insurers' schemes to supplementary insurance benefits. In 2006, six insurance companies in Croatia offered private (supplementary) health insurance. They mostly contracted private and public health care providers, but some have started to develop networks of providers of their own.

2.3. Announced Changes

According to the proposal of the 2006 Health Care Act, the Croatian Ministry of Health and Social Affairs intends to make an additional step to encourage private health insurance companies to offer Complementary health insurance, in order to decrease the number of subsidized users who procure it from the HZZO.

Should the new law be passed, private insurers will be allowed to combine Complementary health insurance with other existing insurance products, and to offer it through risk rated premiums. While this reform certainly has the potential to attract private health insurers into the Complementary health insurance business, its impact on the social foundations of the insurance system and on the sustainability of the government's (HZZOs) Complementary insurance remain to be seen.

CONCLUSION

It could be argued that the Croatian health care system, although reformed, has retained some of its characteristics from the period of self management. Its legacy from self management includes the powerful voice of the system's users and employees, a strong belief of the public that medical services should be free at the point of use and little regard for the cost of care provided. This has been aggravated by the devastating war imposed on Croatia and the rising numbers of users who do not financially contribute to its treasury, such as the elderly, unemployed, veterans and so on.

Thus, the Croatian health care system, burdened by rising expenditure and financial deficits, balances on the thin line between preserving social justice (or rather social peace) and market reforms. As in other countries, political parties, unions and professionals' and users' organizations, all (naturally) representing their individual interests continuously shift the debate from policy to politics.

However, in order to preserve its sustainability, the system will require substantial reforms based on evidence and analysis, rather than, as was the case so far, those based on power relations and the struggle for citizens' votes in political elections.

REFERENCES:

1. Šaric M, Rodwin V. G, The once and future health system in the former Yugoslavia: myths and realities. *J Public Health Policy* 1993; 14: 220-3
2. Letica S. *Zdravstvena politika u doba krize.* Zagreb: Naprijed, 1989.
3. Hebrang A. Reorganization of the Croatian health care system. *Croatian Med J* 1994; 35: 130-136
4. HIT (Health Care System in Transition) *Croatia:* European Observatory on Health Care Systems, World Health Organization, Regional Office for Europe; 1999.
5. Kovacic L, Sosic Z. Organization of Health Care in Croatia: Needs and Priorities. *Croatian Med J.* 1998; 39: (3).
6. Hebrang A, Njavro J, Mrkonji? I. Komentar Zakona o Zdravstvenoj zaštiti i Zdravstvnom osiguranju. Zagreb: Privredni biro, 1993.
7. Ministry of Health and Social Care, National Strategy for the Development of Health Care from 2006-2011, Zagreb 2006
8. Croatian Institute for Health Insurance. Financial report for year 2003; Zagreb, 2004 www.hzzo-net.hr
9. Croatian Institute for Health Insurance. Financial report for year 2002. Godisnje izvjesce o poslovanju zdravstvenog osiguranja i zdravstva Republike Hrvatske za 2002. godinu [in Croatian] Zagreb; 2003 www.hzzo-net.hr
10. World Health Organization. *The World Health Report 2005: Make Every Mother and Child Count,* Statistical annex; 2005
11. Mastilica M, Bozikov J. Out-of-pocket payments for Health Care in Croatia: implications for equity. *Croatian Medical Journal* 1999; 40(2): 152-9
12. Lewis M. Informal Health Payments in Central and Eastern Europe and the Former Soviet Union: Issues, Trends and Policy Implications in Mossialos E, Dixon A, Figueras J, Kutzin J (editors) *Funding Health Care: Options for Europe.* Buckingham: Open University Press; 2002
13. World Bank Europe and Central Asia Region, Human Development Department. Croatia Health Finance Study. World Bank, Washington, D.C.; 2004 online http://www-wds.worldbank.org/servlet/WDS_IBank_Servlet?pcont=details&eid=00001 2009_20040616103200 Accessed on 20 February 2005.

A new prevention law in Germany: Change of paradigm, increased bureaucracy – or both?

Rolf Rosenbrock

1. The epidemiological situation in Germany and its political consequences

The epidemiological situation in Germany resembles that of other industrialized countries: Morbidity and mortality are dominated by a few chronic degenerative illnesses known as the "big killers" (coronary heart disease, cancer etc.) and the "big cripplers" (musculo-skeletal disorders, diabetes, chronic obstructive pulmonary disease, depression, alcohol and drug dependency). Costs incurred for the care of patients suffering from these illnesses consume three quarters of health expenditures. Theoretically, a large part of these illnesses could be prevented. It is impossible to give a sound estimate of how large this part might be. In Germany, a popular, but controversial study suggests that a quarter of the disease burden might be prevented.

At the same time, life expectancy is increasing by more than one year per decade. This does not, however, mean a continual rise in the number of years sick; due to the compression of morbidity, people are remaining healthier in their later years. A maximum of one third of these improvements can be attributed to clinical medicine. A minimum of two thirds can be explained by an improvement in living conditions and education, which in turn generate healthier behaviour. That is, at least two thirds of the health improvements observed are the result of social developments and are therefore due to implicit health policy. It would be interesting to know how much planned prevention measures (explicit health policy) has contributed towards these health improvements. I do not know of any sound empirical investigations into this question.

Another tendency – also due to implicit health policy inherent in labour market, educational and social policy etc. –are the growing inequalities in health in Germany. The life expectancy of men from the lowest 25 % in terms of income is about ten years shorter than that of men from the highest 25 %. For women this difference amounts to about five years. In addition, the socially disadvantaged experience more years of chronic illness and disability. At all stages of their lives – from the cradle to the grave – people from the lowest 20 % according to socio-economic status run double the risk of falling seriously ill or dying prematurely as compared to persons in the highest 20 %. Primary prevention in health policy, therefore, has to aim at extending the compression of morbidity to include people of lower socioeconomic status.

In spite of generally having equal access to qualitatively good health care, the chronically ill on the lower rungs of the social ladder are on average less well taken care of than the economically better off. These inequities are mostly due to the poor organisation of health care, particularly with regard to the coordination and integration of care provided by general practitioners, specialists, and inpatient treatment. The lack of integration of medical care, nursing, and social work services as well as the failing coordination of self-help and professional services are further factors contributing to the problem.

That the "inverse care law" described by Tudor Hart in 1971 also applies to Germany in spite of the existence of social health insurance is mostly due to the fact that the burden of care integration has been passed on to the patients. Thus, people with lower levels of education and social capital are structurally disadvantaged. This does not imply an absolute impoverishment of the lower social strata; their life expectancy is increasing as well, but at a slower pace as compared to the better-off and as compared to the average for the population as a whole. The number of poor people continues to rise in Germany even under a social democratic-green government (currently 13.5 % of the population, according to the EU-definition).

The results of an international comparison of education systems and outcomes (PISA) show that the German system of education does not promote upward mobility of the socially disadvantaged as strongly as it could. Given these tendencies, there is little hope that social differences with regard to health and life expectancy will decrease in the foreseeable future.

For researchers in public health and others promoting a stronger explicit health policy this situation presents three primary challenges:

It is necessary to point out time and again that neo-liberal policies at all levels create more health problems – thereby increasing health care costs – than explicit health policy is able to cope with. I would not claim that society should be shaped solely according to the needs of a health-based public policy. Most of us would not want to live in such a society. I would also not set absolute equality as the goal. Rather, we are talking about an equality of opportunity.

The question is: How much inequality does a society need in order to supply sufficient incentives for achievement and innovation? And how much equality does a society need in order to rightfully pass as "civilized"? In this debate the health sciences have to make themselves heard more clearly. The fact that, with a time lag from three to four years, labour market and education policies also affect a population's health, is often overlooked as is the scope of socially caused inequality in health and other outcomes, more generally.

The second challenge consists in providing integrated care, safeguarding patients' dignity, and considering social factors in the organisation of care, especially for the chronically ill. To fill in more details on this point would take us too far afield.

I would like to focus on the third challenge we face, which is how to maximize the preventive potential in existing structures. This topic will be discussed more thoroughly in light of current developments in Germany.

2. The state of the art in primary prevention

Based on years of experience we know that effective prevention is characterized by the following four features:

a. Reduction of health burdens and promotion of resources

In some cases, it may be sufficient to focus on health burdens in order to achieve better health outcomes– as for example on environmental stressors, poor nutrition, smoking, lack of exercise, or social isolation. In general, however, it is more appropriate to focus on promoting health resources at the individual and group level – self-esteem, self-efficacy, life skills, and information seeking. Such strategies aim at:

● increasing the physical and psychological potential of coping with health burdens;

● strengthening the individual capacity to overcome risk behaviour;

● expanding competencies for structural change in order to minimize health burdens.

b. Revaluating non-specific interventions

The history of successful primary prevention shows that one and the same strategy – for example urban renewal or improvements in an education system,. – can contribute to the reduction of several different illnesses simultaneously. The same effect can also be observed with regard to integrated strategies of worksite health promotion (Lenhardt et al. 1997; Lenhardt 2003). The impact of interventions addressing so-called "distal causes" of disease such as community mobilization and social support has not yet been sufficiently examined. Experience shows, however, that addressing distal social causes may have greater preventive effects on a population's morbidity and mortality rate than focussing solely on biological proximal causes. This also holds true for the alleviation of health burdens, more generally, as well as for the strengthening of health resources.

c. Priority of addressing context

In order to reach the best possible prevention results with regard to socially disadvantaged groups interventions should not be limited to the instruments of information, education, and counselling. Chances for success are much better when the behavioural context is addressed – on the individual level, in settings (a concept which in Germany designates both community-based interventions as well as those confined to a particular location) and within the framework of integrated, multimodal, and intersectoral campaigns targeting the population in general or defined subgroups.

As interventions restricted to information, education, and counselling are less complex, less expensive, and provoke fewer conflicts among stakeholders they are usually easier to push through, in spite of the fact that they are generally less effective and sustainable. Interventions addressing contextual factors and aimed at changing them usually encounter stronger political opposition (Kühn/Rosenbrock 1994).

d. Priority of participation

Paolo Freire's practical and theoretical work of the late 1970s demonstrated that people with little formal education are most successful at learning new concepts and behaviours if such learning is linked to their everyday lives and if they are able to practice what they have learned in their daily environment (Freire 1980).

The leading example of successful primary prevention in a specific setting, worksite health promotion, has made clear that changes of behaviour and attitudes are successful and sustainable to the degree which the employees are involved in needs assessment, planning, implementation, and evaluation of change efforts (Wright 2004). From this experience follows the demand for a high degree of direct participation of the target groups in designing and implementing interventions..

Strategies for primary prevention focussing on the reduction of health burdens and the promotion of health resources can be implemented on three levels: the individual, the setting or community, and the general population. Interventions can be further classified based on whether they are confined to information, education, and counselling or whether they also address contextual factors. An example for each of these types is given in figure 1.

Each of these strategy types requires different tools, resources, constellations of players, and methods of quality assurance(1). It is a central task of health policy and management to make sure that the appropriate type of strategy is used, depending on health risk and target group. The usual political tendency is to take recourse to less complex types of intervention (e. g. individual instead of setting interventions) even where more complex interventions are indicated. The measure of all political attempts to improve prevention is the degree to which they succeed on countering this tendency.

3. A new prevention law in Germany

In 2005 the 'Law on the improvement of health prevention' (Gesetz zur Stärkung der gesundheitlichen Prävention) will take effect in Germany, thus making prevention the "fourth pillar" of the health care system, the

Figure 1: Types of primary prevention

	Information, education, counselling	Context-based
Individual	1. e. g. prevention information from a primary care physician, health courses	2. e. g. preventive home visits
Setting/ Community	3. e. g. anti-tobacco education in schools	4. e. g. worksite health promotion as organizational development
General population	5. e. g. 'Eat more fruit' 'Physical exercise is good for you' 'Smoking is hazardous to your health'	6. e. g. HIV/AIDS campaign, exercise campaigns

other three pillars being curative medicine, nursing care, and rehabilitation. This law is the culmination of four different strands of development over the last several years (Rosenbrock 2004c):

In 2001 the federal government invited all relevant players of the health care system to a series of round table discussions on the key problems of health policy. In the field of prevention this led to the emergence of the 'German Forum on Prevention and Health Promotion' (Deutsches Forum Prävention und Gesundheitsförderung) which became a permanent organisational platform to formulate new programmes involving some 60 participants interested in prevention (professional associations, NGOs, various state institutions, etc.).

These activities were flanked by official statements from the German Parliament (Bundestag and Bundesrat), the trade unions, employers' associations, political parties and other bodies demanding a strengthening of structures and resources for primary prevention.

At the same time, after a long period of discussion between professional associations, NGOs , researchers, and government representatives, the federally funded project to set health goals at the national level (gesundheitsziele.de) formulated a number of health targets and priorities. (BMGS 2003).

Already in 1989 the health insurers in Germany had been commissioned to organize primary prevention activities on a smaller scale.. These activities were stopped in 1996 as the conflicts in providing such services became apparent. The insurance providers had readily taken up the topic of primary prevention and were able to produce major successful innovations particularly in the field of worksite health promotion. Their endeavours did, however, bear the mark of the contradictory demands they had to meet.

Due to economic competition insurers were more interested in "good risks" (so-called 'cherry picking'), whereas their prevention efforts were to be directed primarily towards the poor. In most cases, economic incentives proved to be stronger. Insurance providers mainly organised health training courses for the middle class while preventive interventions in socially disadvantaged settings (schools, neighbourhoods etc.) were neglected. Thus, the expectation that primary prevention undertaken by insurance providers could meet the needs of the poor proved to be unrealistic.

After a period of negotiation with social insurance representatives (particularly health insurers) and state governments (Länder), the federal government published in the fall of 2004 an outline for a proposed prevention law including the following points:

Primary prevention services provided by government authorities (e.g.local public health authorities) are not to be diminished or replaced, but rather augmented by new money from social insurance funds and not from tax revenue. This decision was fiscally motivated.

It was argued that social insurance providers were already involved in the field of prevention (Walter 2003) and that their scope of action could not be reduced to the administration of benefits in the case of need. Although this argument does not exclude the use of tax revenue for financing prevention, the decision finally taken favours the participation of all social insurers in all stages of the decision process and therefore generates a considerable demand for negotiation and consensus, which might lead to a loss of innovative strength and efficiency.

In view of the likelihood that health inequalities in Germany are growing, the law would link primary prevention to the main target of reducing these inequalities as well as inequalities based on gender.

Primary prevention funded by health insurers according to §20 of the 5th Book of the Social Code proved to be heavily biased towards measures focusing on attitudes and behaviours instead of contextual factors. This problem would be tackled by fixing a minimum proportion of 40 % of all expenditures on primary prevention to be spent on setting projects and programmes rooted in the everyday life of the socially disadvantaged.

Both centralised and de-centralised structures are foreseen for the administration of prevention. Decisions regarding specific interventions are decentralised. Issues of overarching targets for prevention interventions as well as for quality assurance will be managed by a centralised structure. The law will try to meet these requirements by creating three levels of decision.

Like in Switzerland, this newly created structure centres around a foundation financed by insurance contributions to compulsory health insurance (pension insurance, accident insurance, and long-term care insurance schemes) in cooperation with the federal states (Länder) and the local authorities. The funds of this foundation are to be used to finance and implement prevention measures. The social insurance providers and the foundation are called 'social agents of prevention' in the proposed the law.

Uniform definitions of primary, secondary and tertiary prevention as well as health promotion will be formulated. Also, forms of intervention, quality assurance and intervention targets will be defined. These will be applied to three levels of primary prevention related activities:

At the federal level there will a foundation funded by the health, pension, work accident and long-term care insurers. This foundation will fulfil coordinating tasks. These include the formulation and recommendation of health targets, the organisation of campaigns, implementation pilot projects, as well as the formulation of measures, criteria, and approaches of quality assurance obligatory for all levels of activities. Health targets are to be based on epidemiological data collected and prepared for this purpose by the Robert Koch Institute (RKI), Germany's centre for disease control and surveillance. The national campaigns will draw directly on the expertise and resources of the Federal Centre for Health Education (Bundeszentrale für gesundheitliche Aufklärung).

At the state level community/setting-based projects will be implemented, financed by the health, pension, work accident, and long-term care insurers.

At the level of the individual social insurers (health, pension, work accident, and long-term care) activities will be carried out to influence health attitudes and behaviours through various courses as well as through worksite health promotion. The financing of worksite health promotion does not directly fit into the terms of the prevention law, but rather represents a concession to the insurers who wanted to keep a competitive edge by being able to offer their own package of prevention interventions for their members.

From 2005 to 2007 the financing of these structures will continuously rise until the full amount of EUR 250 million is reached in 2008. Of these funds the foundation is to receive EUR 50 million, and a total of EUR 100 million is to be turned over to the decision-making bodies created at the state level. This leaves EUR 100 million for the social insurance providers who will continue to organise their own prevention courses, etc. within the framework of set targets and quality assurance.

The total of EUR 250 million consists of EUR 180 million from compulsory health insurance whose expenditures on prevention will thereby decrease by 20 per cent. This is compared to the amount of some EUR 2.64 per head of the 70 million insured in 2003 which the insurers were authorised to spend according to the former legislation (§20 SGB V), although this sum was never fully spent.

Of the EUR 180 million, EUR 36 million will be turned over to the foundation, EUR 72 million to the decision-making bodies on the state level and another EUR 72 million Euros will be go to the prevention courses and worksite health promotion implemented directly by the health insurers.

The compulsory pension scheme will contribute a total of EUR 40 million which will be diverted from the funds formerly spent on rehabilitation (tertiary prevention). Of this money the foundation will receive EUR 8 million; EUR 16 million each are to be spent on setting projects at the state level and on prevention courses organised by the pension insurers themselves.

The compulsory work-related accident insurance scheme will contribute EUR 20 million, EUR 4 million of which will go to the foundation and EUR 8 million each are to be spent on worksite setting projects and on prevention courses. This leaves more than 90 per cent of the total contributed by accident insurers for primary prevention (amounting to some EUR 700 million) outside the regulatory framework of the prevention law. The long-term care insurance will pay a total of ten million Euros, two million of which go to the foundation and four million each are to be spent on setting projects and prevention courses.

As the federal government is not authorised to regulate the use of funds raised by private health and private long-term care insurances, these companies will be asked to make voluntary contributions to the implementation of the prevention law. Due to political differences between the Federal Ministry of Health and Social Security (BMGS) and the Federal Ministry of Economics and Labour (BMWA), the Federal Employment Agency responsible for unemployment insurance (SGB III) has not yet been integrated into the structures of the law, although the Agency's clients – more than 5 million officially registered unemployed in Germany – are affected most acutely by inequalities in health. Those who have been unemployed for more than 12 months run double the risk of morbidity and mortality as compared to the working population. The participation of unemployment insurance in the funding of primary prevention will therefore remain a contentious issue.

Assessing the law

The 'Law on the improvement of health prevention' will create a very complex structure with a host of decision-making bodies and competencies typical of the German ('corporatistic') system of governance by associations ('path dependency'). From a health policy point of view the following traits can be seen as positive:

● The (modest) increase of resources for primary prevention;

● The significant increase in resources for setting projects;

● The integration of campaigns addressing the general population into the repertoire of primary prevention tools;

● The mandatory orientation of primary prevention towards science-based health targets;

● The requirement of primary prevention to reduce inequalities of health caused by social status and gender;

● The mandatory setting of standards for quality assurance, as well as

● The integration of pension, accident, and long-term care insurance in the funding mechanism.

Whether the complex negotiation processes will lead to the measures envisaged by health policy experts remains an open question. Doubts are being raised based on the fact that the foundation is only authorised to recommend targets etc. (§ 11 section 1). There is a clause in the law which will allow the states (§ 12 section 3) as well as social security providers (§ 17 section 6) to sidestep centrally fixed targets and programmes. Another problem is that the foundation needs the consent of the decision-making bodies at the state level.

On the whole it remains to be seen whether the cross-level instruments of coordination are sufficient to curb the autonomous interests of the 'social agents of prevention'. It is quite obvious that the changing federal governments will try to make use of national health campaigns for their own purposes, such interventions requiring the coordination of health messages in the mass media, in setting projects as well as in individual-oriented prevention courses.

On the state level there is a permanent interest in expanding the grossly underfinanced sector of public health services by using the funds provided by the prevention law. Without adequate controls over the forces of competition (such as risk-compensation schemes), health insurers will continue to be more interested in optimizing their risk-pools than in orienting prevention courses toward a reduction of health inequalities.

In view of all these diverging interests and incentives it is not clear whether the prevention law will succeed in turning primary prevention into a strong 'pillar' of health protection. The success will depend on the extent to which all parties involved actually strive toward the goal of improving the public's health. If the regulatory approach grounded in the prevention law serves its purpose, it will probably only be a few years time before the question arises as to whether the financial means set aside for primary prevention – amounting to approximately two thousandths of health care expenditures – is sufficient.

---

[1] Each of these six strategy types, if conducted according to international standards, addresses both the reduction of health burdens (prevention in the narrow sense) as well as the strengthening of health resources (health promotion).

Changes in Drug Approval in the EU and Germany: from regulation to service

Rolf Schmucker

Introduction

Drug approval in Germany is about to undergo far-reaching changes. The major political parties agree that the approval procedure should be made faster and more efficient. In April 2005, the Federal Government passed a bill, which is intended to put drug approval on a new footing in Germany. In future, the German agency for drugs and medical products, DAMA, is to take the place of the federal institute for drugs and medical products, BfArM.

The impending restructuring of drugs approval goes beyond organisational innovations. With this, the character of the approval authority is changed profoundly. The theory proclaimed here says that German national drugs approval is going to change from a national regulatory body of the pharmaceutical industry to a service agency for the pharmaceutical industry, which is based on commercial criteria.

This development can however not only be observed in Germany. It is being performed throughout the entire EU and is characterised by European jurisdiction on drugs approval. An interaction of national and European levels is the result, in which the increased pressure is put on national approval agencies to conform. Speed and efficiency of the approval process is the prime target, not least in the interest of the competitiveness of the European pharmaceutical industry with their North American competitors.

Drugs approval is an example of the immediate impact of the European process of integration on national health systems. By using

Germany as an example, we are going to show the process of interaction of regulation at European and at national levels. For this purpose, we will first show an outline of the European dimension of drugs approval. The second step will then describe the development in Germany. Finally, we are going to evaluate the changes taking place in drugs approval, identifying the risks they bring in train.

1. The European level

Since 1975, the EU has been trying without success to implement an effective European standardisation of drugs approval (see Permanand & Mossialos 2004). The project of the common European market and the subsequent internationalisation of the pharmaceutical market was a strong incentive for these efforts. In 1993, a European standard of drugs approval was finally achieved (VO (EWG) 2309/93), which quickly became significant. By introducing the EMEA (European Medicinal Evaluation Agency), a European agency for the approval was created, which provided an important precondition for a standardised European regulation. Since 1995, two different methods of approval have been existing at a European level: the Centralised Procedure (CP) and the Mutual Recognition Procedure (MRP).

The Centralised Procedure is compulsory for innovative bio-technological medicines and an optional process for other innovative preparations. The basic innovation was that decisions regarding the approval of drugs were made by a central European institution on behalf of the entire EU region. The CP mainly serves the interests of research intensive, internationally oriented businesses and is to bolster European industry as an innovative force and as a place of research and production. The procedure represents the largest step so far in the direction of a europeanisation of drugs approval. It is characterised on one hand, by the final say being at a European level, and on the other hand, by the integration of the national evaluation agencies and registration bodies into the evaluation and decision-making process.

Within the EMEA, this evaluation committee (CPMP1: Committee for Proprietary Medicinal Products), which consists of two representatives each of the national regulation agencies, is responsible for devising evaluative recommendations. For this, reports are produced by two members of the CPMP (reporter, co-reporter), based on the assessments of external experts and with the support of their relevant national authorities. The EMEA pass the resulting recommendation to the commission, who produce the draft of a decision. This will be decided – by qualified majority – by the standing committee, which consists of representatives of the national governments. The decision of approval is pronounced by the commission. In the event of a rejection by the standing committee – which has not happened so far – the council of ministers will become involved (see Feick 2002b: 15ff.).

The Mutual Recognition Procedure is open to drugs that are to be marketed in more than one EU member state (does not apply to innovative biotechnological preparations). The national authorities remain the authorities for implementation. On the face of it, the MRP resembles the old multi-state procedure; it however contains a "structural step of europeanisation" in that it intends to include binding arbitration proceedings at a European level (which it however does not prescribe as compulsory). It is suitable for different categories of drugs (and companies), depending on their strategic orientation. It shows fewer European centralised components, which are also not applied very often.

The flexibility of the procedure is appreciated by companies; its efficiency is however much criticised. Applications are made in a Reference Member State (RMS) and in one or several Concerned Member States (CMS). The authority of the RMS produces the drafts for evaluation and decision, the authority of the CMS has the right to approve or to reject these. In the event of disputes, two trans-national stages can be used; an arbitration meeting of the two involved players and arbitration between the players involved, with the involvement of the EMEA, the commission and the council of ministers (like in the Centralised Procedure) (see Feick 2002b: 19ff.).

The revision of the European approval procedures in 2004 (VO (EG) 726/2004) expanded and strengthened the proceedings. The group of drugs for which approval by the CP is obligatory was expanded (new active ingredients for the treatment of AIDS, cancer, neurodegenerative conditions, diabetes; from 2008 onwards: auto-immune diseases, other immune deficiencies, viral diseases). In addition to this, a fast-track process has been introduced, i.e. an accelerated evaluation procedure for human medicines, which "are of interest to public health and particularly under the aspect of therapeutic innovations" (§14, sub-section 9). For medication which meets these standards, the procedural period is reduced from 210 to 150 days.

The introduction of the European procedures in 1995 has fundamentally altered the standards for the approval of drugs. Now, there is a range of approval proceedings for manufacturers of pharmaceutical products from which they are able to choose – depending on their specific product range and their marketing strategy. This has far-reaching consequences for national authorities. The MRP immediately puts the various national agencies into a position of competition. In the CP, the significance of the national agency depends on whether it has been selected to be the reporter or co-reporter. This has not only an impact on the reputation of this authority but also the situation regarding orders and finances and thus also on its existence. The strong influence which the interests of the pharmaceutical industry has on European approval policies has incited criticism. The measures, which Li Bassi (among others) suggested in 2003, with the help of which the needs and interests of the patients were to receive absolute priority at all levels of the approval process, were however not taken into account in the revision of 2004.

2. Drugs approval in Germany

Until 1978, there was no national procedure for the approval of drugs. Medication launched on the market was usually only registered by the federal health authority (BGA). The BGA consequently also was not authorised to reject the registration if a hazardous effect of the drug was suspected. Only the passing in 1978 of the act restructuring the law on drugs caused an approval process to be introduced, in which the quality, effectiveness and the innocuousness of drugs were demanded as test criteria. Medication, which had been introduced on the market before 1978, is tested in a subsequent approval or subsequent registration procedure (see Murswieck 1983: 284ff.). In 1994, the federal institute for drugs and medical products (BfArM) took on the task of drugs approval. This is an independent senior federal authority in the ambit of the federal ministry for health and social security (BMGS) (see BfArM 2005).

The core duties of the BfArM consist of the approval and the registration of drugs and the risk monitoring of already approved drugs (pharmacological vigilance). The federal opium agency at the institute regulates and controls the legal use of narcotics. In addition to this, the BfArM is the registration office for risks incurring in the use of medicines. The legal basis of the approval proceedings can be found in the drugs act (AMG), which defines its purpose in §1: "to provide safety in the handling of drugs, particularly regarding the quality, effectiveness and innocuousness of medicines (...)". Ready-to-use drugs, i.e. "drugs, which have been produced in advance and are circulated in a package designed for the user" (§4, sub-section 1 AMG), are subject to the obligation of approval, i.e. they must either be approved by the authority responsible (the BfArM) or by the European Council or the European Commission (§21). Approval is to be applied for by the pharmaceutical company.

The application should include a number of approval documents, which as a rule must include information regarding the name of the drug, its components, its effects, fields of application, contraindication, etc. In addition to this, all results of analytical, pharmacological-toxicological and clinical tests, which are relevant for the evaluation of the drug, must be presented.

This both includes favourable and unfavourable information on the drug (§22, sub-section 1.2 AMG). In connection with the Centralised European proceedings, the BfArM is able to act as reporter or as co-reporter.

2.1. Criticism of the German approval procedure

For a few years, the BfArM has been receiving criticism from various sides. This particularly concerns the speed and the efficiency of the approval proceedings:

● Duration of proceedings: the average duration, especially if the national approval proceedings are too long. The statutory standard of the duration of the proceedings is 7 months (§27 AMG). Currently, the average is 26 months. However, this does not apply to the European proceedings into which the BfArM is integrated, and which show a shorter procedural duration.

● The proportion of European approval proceedings: statistically, Germany is only fifth in Europe (after the UK, Sweden, the Netherlands and Denmark). This is said to be too little for the country with the largest pharmaceutical market.

● Opportunities for co-operation: it is said that the authority does not co-operate sufficiently with the applicants. The ban on contacts prior to the submission of the application has been particularly criticised. Instead, companies should be able to discuss the crucial points of the proceedings with the authority, which should be able to advise them.

In 2003, the BMGS introduced a "Taskforce for the improvement of the conditions of the location and opportunities for innovation of the German pharmaceutics industry", which consisted of representatives of the federal ministry for health, the ministry of finance, the pharmaceutical industry, the trade union for chemical workers, as well as the business consultants Boston Consulting Group.

This Taskforce underpinned the previously named points of criticism and demanded faster and more efficient approval proceedings. Greater efficiency was said to require "a new identity for its (the federal agency, R.S.) role as the partner in the interaction of industry, science and patients" and the Taskforce continued:

"The role model of the agency should among other things be an attitude, which is fundamentally positive and favourable regarding innovation."

The restructuring is regarded as the most important basic requirement for the marketing of products produced in Germany. In addition to this, this should be a source of new impetus for the pharmaceutical industry, ensuring export opportunities for the manufacturers of medicines, "who are able to use the approval by a recognised authority as an advertising bonus" (see Taskforce 2004). Specifically, the Taskforce produced an action plan, which intends a number of measures for drugs approval. These mainly concerned the improvement of the efficiency of the BfArM with streamlined project management, clearly defined responsibilities, greater transparency and better information. The situation of the authority when competing against other approval authorities was to be improved with a larger number of competent staff. A greater independence regarding the budget was to increase the flexibility of the authority. At EU level, the agency was to work towards a reduction of the administrative effort and a simplification of procedures.

In 2004 an evaluation report was also issued by the science council (Wissenschaftsrat), which advises the government on issues of universities, science and research. Although the science council testifies that the BfArM was committed and used a large number of staff, it also criticised the agency for still being "unable to show the same efficiency as other approval agencies abroad." (Wissenschaftsrat 2004: 67).

It was said that the lack of internal research conducted was a particular deficiency, which had an influence on the standard of scientific expertise. The science council demanded a restructuring of the BfArM, in connection with this, their research base was to be expanded. The introduction of a research director, the opening of a research budget and the formulation of a consistent research programme are significant steps, with which the profile within the European approval environment could be defined more clearly.

"With the deliberate development of a field of research, which is of particular interest at a European level, the BfArM was to develop into an internationally recognised centre of competence with exclusive characteristics" (ibid.: 67f.).

2.2. The bill for the development of a German drugs agency

In April 2005, the German government decided on the bill on the restructuring of the approval agency DAMA (DAMA Development Act). The replacement of the BfArM by DAMA, which was to be completed by 2006, had the aim "to ensure effective approval management at a high scientific level for the area of drugs approval. This requires an organisational reform, which is characterised by flexible service management based on international standards, which enable fast and qualified decisions" (Bundesregierung 2005).

As justification for the revision of the drugs approval system, the government cited international competition within the pharmaceutical industry ... and the European competition between approval agencies. In this "dual competition", the major aim is the acceleration of the proceedings, which should be both in the interest of the pharmaceutical industry and the patient. It was also to improve the position of the authority vis a vis its European competitors.

These aims were to be achieved with a fundamental restructuring of the approval authority. The legal form of the authority is changed from a supreme federal authority to a government office. This causes DAMA to have greater autonomy than its predecessor. The federal ministry for health and social security would no longer be able to exercise an unlimited right to issue instructions but it would exercise a supervisory function regarding the "legitimacy of the execution of tasks", as well as the right "to issue general qualified instructions" (ibid.: 32).

DAMA was to receive independence regarding its organisation, staff and finances. The supervisory board, which was to consist of two members, was not to have the status of civil servants but should be subject to a private employment relationship and should thus support the "flexible and modern" service management of the agency. Following criticism of the science council and the task force, the substance of the bill demands "the abandonment of the current orientation, which is typical for public offices," and "a greater market orientation" of the federal institute, "as has already been performed in other countries" (ibid.: 30).

A change is also intended in the financing of DAMA. The government intends largely to withdraw from the financing of the agency. For the area of drugs approval, the principle of self-financing should be applied, i.e. the activities of DAMA should be completely financed through the fees and payments of the applicants. For the area of risk monitoring of approved drugs (pharmacological vigilance) and of medical products, which are not immediately connected to drugs approval, financing with tax revenue should be possible. The right to receive government funds is however only granted to DAMA "if its total revenue would not be sufficient to cover its expenses without government funding. This would take into account the aim that the financing of the German drugs agency should as far as possible be carried out without government funds" (ibid: 42).

3. Outlook: from regulating authority to service agency

Following the Thalidomide catastrophe of the early 1960s (in Germany, this drug was approved under the name of Contergan), intense discussions regarding necessary reforms of drugs approval ensued, and not only in the EU. At the forefront was the criterion of consumer or patient protection and thus the question of how such catastrophes can be avoided in future. The tendency was to strengthen the competencies of the national regulatory authorities and to intensify their controlling functions. The orientation of the debate has since changed, and this is both apparent in the European regulation and in the present bill for the introduction of DAMA.

To strengthen the compatibility of the pharmaceutics industry becomes an elementary target of the approval proceedings. Here, the speed, with which a new drug can be launched on the market, plays a significant part. The result of fast approval is a major commercial gain for the company in question. Depending on the product and the target market, the European diversification of the approval methods makes it possible to choose the most suitable proceedings, as well as the place of approval.

This is favourable for the different sizes of businesses, product ranges and marketing strategies. The national agencies are under increased pressure to present themselves to the applicants as quickly and efficiently acting agencies. In addition to this, the co-operation with the public authorities is also of great importance to the industry. A close co-operation – even prior to application – would contribute to solving problems at an early stage.

In the long term, the pressure of international competition on the pharmaceutical market will only allow authorities to survive if they are able to match the ideas of the industry regarding efficiency. The German approval agency is competing with 41 other agencies in the enlarged EU. The tendency is to reduce the number of relevant European agencies to only a few centres of competence. Germany has the largest market for drugs in Europe; statistically, it is however only fifth in the number of approvals. The increase in efficiency, which is the aim of the present bill, is to redress this balance.

The German government intends to use this to bolster Germany as a site for the pharmaceutical industry. This both applies to the area of research and development and production. Under the conditions of European and global competition, the work of the approval agency is considered to be a decisive factor. By the same token, this bill is going to fundamentally change the character of the authority. The underlying principle of the revision is to rebuilt the authority into a modern, efficient and competitive service agency.

The changes as described above are linked to risks, which particularly concern the issue of drug safety. The following section is going to discuss three basic risks: the clash of interests of approval agency and industry, the possible consequences of financing through fees, as well as the risks deriving from the acceleration of proceedings.

The bias in drug regulation in favour of the interests of the pharmaceutical industry, which Abraham and Lewis diagnosed for the European proceedings in 2000, is illustrated by the DAMA introduction act. Guiding the applicant through the proceedings as fast and as efficiently as possible is going to become DAMA's central principle for action. The complexity of this matter and the proceedings require close co-operation between the regulators and those who are regulated, and in this arena the industry has the larger financial means and organisational resources. Compared to this, the ability to organise and mobilise consumer interests is significantly smaller. There is a danger that the regulatory authority is taken over by the industry, thus losing its ability and its incentive to control (see Feick 2002a: 28).

The clash of interests of agency and industry is made worse by the increasing importance of the financing through fees. The government withdraws from its responsibilities. The effectiveness of the authority thus hangs in the balance. Even if pharmacological vigilance were to continue to be financed by tax funds, it seems doubtful that DAMA will be able to retain its independence in the delicate area of risk assessment of approved drugs. A conflict between institutional interests and the legal responsibility of the authority is looming on the horizon. When it comes to deciding how the risks of a drug should be evaluated, the orientation of the agency to its industry "customers" is in potential opposition to its statutory mandate to "provide safety regarding the handling of drugs" (§1 AMG).

Those who approve of the restructuring of the authority argue that the safety of drugs is an inherent interest of the manufacturer and that a loss of quality is therefore not to be expected. This is also claimed for the intended acceleration of the proceedings. The experience of past years however shows that, in the area of tension between commercial interests and safety, the former often receives preference.

This can be demonstrated by showing the development of the US Food and Drugs Administration (FDA). At the beginning of the 1990s, the FDA had achieved a reduction of the approval period from 21 to 12 months. In fast track proceedings, this is even reduced to six months. The quota of approved drugs has increased from 60 to 80%. However, at the same time, the instances of unwanted side effects have increased – and between 1997 and 2000, 14 products were recalled (Kiewel 2003: 13).

A report of the health committee of the British House of Commons also takes a critical view on the importance of the acceleration of proceedings.

> "Our inquiry revealed major failings in the regulatory system. The organisation, process and techniques of the MHRA are focussed on bringing drugs to market fast. The stated rationale, that patients benefit from new drugs, is insufficiently qualified by considerations of relative merit or value, or therapeutic need" (House of Commons/Health Committee 2005: 103).

The British discussion also sees the competition between European approval agencies as a factor that reduces the influence of patient protection in the approval proceedings (ibid.: 106).

The risks to the health of patients, however, which often arise from modern, highly effective drugs however increase the need for independent governmental control of the pharmaceutical market.

> "If patients' interests are to be defended, then the drugs that are approved must be rigorously evaluated and demonstrate comparative benefit. For this to become reality, [an authorization agency] must become a strong organisation, with adequate resources to meet the challenges posed by the pharmaceutical industry" (Garattini/Bertele 2004: 94).

The changes in the regulatory system planned in Germany however point into a different direction.

Note

(1) In 2004, the revision of the proceedings replaced directive (EWG) no. 2309/93 by regulation (EG) no. 726/2004. This resulted in a few names of institutions involved to be changed. EMEA now stands for European Medicines Agency. The CPMP is now called CHMP (Committee for Medicinal Products for Human Use). This committee is also responsible for pharmacological vigilance, which includes the monitoring of (unwanted) side effects of approved drugs and the renewal of the approval after five years. In the event of serious reactions, the CPMP has the right to issue special warnings or to withdraw the drug from the market.(Garattini/Bertele 2004: 85).

References

Abraham, John / Lewis, G. (2000), Regulating Medicines in Europe: competition, expertise and public health, London/New York.

AMG (Gesetz über den Verkehr mit Arzneimitteln) in der Fassung der Bekanntmachung vom 11. Dezember 1998 (BGBL. I S. 3586); zuletzt geändert durch Art. 2 des Gesetzes vom 10. Februar 2005 (BGBL. I S. 234).

BfArM (Bundesinstitut für Arzneimittel und Medizinprodukte)(2005), Selbstdarstellung, www.bfarm.de/DasBfArM/aufg/index.php am 02.06.2005.

Bundesregierung (2005), Entwurf eines Gesetzes zur Errichtung einer Deutschen Arzneimittelagentur (DAMA-Errichtungsgesetz), http://www.bmgs.bund.de/download/gesetze/entwuerfe/DAMA_Errichtungs gesetz.pdf am 02.05.2005.

Feick, Jürgen (2002a), Der Interessenbezug der europäischen Arzneimittelzulassung, unveröff. Manuskript, MPIfG Köln.

Feick, Jürgen (2002b), Regulatory Europeanization, National Autonomy and Regulatory Effectiveness: Marketing Authorization for Pharmaceuticals, MPIfG Discussion Paper 02/6, November 2002, Köln.

Garratini, Silvio / Bertele, Vittorio (2004), The role of the EMEA in regulating pharmaceutical products, in: Mossialos, Elias / Mrazek, Monique / Walley, Tom (eds.), Regulating pharmaceuticals in Europe: striving for efficiency, equity and quality, Open University Press, Maidenhead, 80-96.

House of Commons/Health Committee (2005), The Influence of the Pharmaceutical Industry. Fourth Report of Session 2004-05, Ordered by The House of Commons to be printed 22 March 2005, London, http://www.publications.parliament.uk/pa/cm200405/cmselect/cmhealth/42/42.pdf am 15.06.2005.

Kiewel, Angelika (2003), Europäische Arzneimittelzulassung im Spagat zwischen Verbrauchersicherheit und Pharmainteressen, in: Die Krankenversicherung, Januar 2003, S. 13-17.

Li Bassi, Luca / Bertele, Vittorio / Garattini, Silvio (2003), European regulatory policies on medicines and public health needs, in: European Journal of

Public Health 2003; 13: 246-251.

Murswieck, Axel (1983), Die staatliche Kontrolle der Arzneimittelsicherheit in der Bundesrepublik und den USA, Opladen.

Permanand, Govin / Mossialos, Elias (2004), Theorising the Development of the European Union Framework for Pharmaceutical Regulation, LSE Health and Social Care Discussion Paper Number 13, London.

Taskforce (2004), Bericht der Taskforce zur Verbesserung der Standortbedingungen und der Innovationsmöglichkeiten der pharmazeutischen Industrie in Deutschland, Berlin 2004, http://www.bmgs.bund.de/download/broschueren/A325.pdf am 17.03.2005

Wissenschaftsrat (2004), Stellungnahme zum Bundesinstitut für Arzneimittel und Medizinprodukte (BfArM), Merseburg, 28. Mai 2004, http://www.wissenschaftsrat.de/texte/6102-04.pdf am 17.03.2005.

Privatisation of health care in Greece: The development of private for-profit health care providers (1980-2002)

Kondilis E,. Giannakopoulos E, Zdoukos T, Gavana M, Benos A

1. Introduction

In Greece, as in most industrialized countries, both provision and financing of health care is based on a public private mix.[1] The National Health System (NHS), founded by the social-democratic government in 1983 following the principles of the Beveridge model, and financed through taxation (mainly indirect taxes), social security payments and users' co-payments, theoretically offers universal coverage to the Greek population.

In parallel, 35 occupational and social security sickness funds, most founded in the early and middle 20th century, financed through proportional contributions from employers and employees, offer coverage to 95% of the population[2], running in some cases their own multi-clinics and few small hospitals.

Finally, private for-profit (PFP) enterprises are involved in both the financing and the provision of health care in Greece. Private health insurance schemes offer duplicate or supplementary coverage to 10% of the population[3], while PFP providers play a constantly ongoing role in the provision of health care services.

The health care system in Greece is deeply fragmented (due to historical reasons[4], reflecting the inborn and structural failures in the

development process of the contemporary Greek State[5]) and characterised by a high level of privatisation. This ongoing process of privatisation in Greece is mainly reflected in the proportionally high levels of
private health expenditure.

In 2001 private health expenditure was estimated between 45.8%
(WHO estimate)[6] and 46.9% (OECD estimate)[7] of total health expenditure. According to the same estimates 95.2% of private health expenditure came from out-of-pocket payments, and only 4.8% from private
health insurance premiums.[6]

Privatisation of health care is based on the conventional wisdom that
the private sector is more efficient and effective than public services[8].
There are three main proposed mechanisms of increasing health care
privatisation[a] rates around the world:

(a) privatisation as a deliberate policy choice, based on the allegation
that a reduction in the role of the state and an increased role for the
private sector is a way to improve resource allocation, efficiency and
quality as well as broaden consumer choice

(b) privatisation as a spontaneous response to poor and inadequate
public health services

(c) privatisation as a response to increased consumer affluence (e.g.
increasing middle-class) and preference for greater quality services.[9]

The present study offers an analysis of the development characteristics of PFP health providers in Greece during the period 1980 – 2002.
This analysis aims at answering the question whether privatisation of
health care in Greece was a spontaneous process due to failures and
"inborn inabilities of public health sector" (passive privatisation) or a
deliberate political choice (incremental privatisation) of both the social-
democratic and conservative governments during the last 25 years.

2. The impact of the foundation of the NHS on private health providers in Greece

Private health care providers have a long tradition in Greek society.
Until the early 1980s the delivery of primary curative services was based
mainly on private physicians, and more than 50% of inpatient care beds
were owned by private for-profit enterprises.[10]

The foundation of the National Health System had a great impact on
the delivery of health care services in Greece. The NHS foundation act
(Law 1397/83) prohibited the establishment, merger or relocation of
private for profit hospitals.[11] Additionally the government kept the

prices, by which the sickness funds compensated the providers for the services consumed by their insured members, at a very low level.[12]

These two factors (the prohibition by the law, and government's adoption of a policy of low prices in health care market) in additional to the rapidly increasing rates of public investment in health care,[13] caused a progressive decline of private for-profit providers (PFP) in Greece during the NHS' implementation period.

Within the next years a great number of clinic owners (especially private consultants owning surgeries with a few beds added on) were forced either to sell their enterprises to the state or convert them into hotels.[14,15]

As it can be seen from the data of the National Statistical Service of Greece both the number of private for-profit hospitals as well as the number of hospital beds owned by the private health sector declined during the decade 1985-1995 (table 1).[16] The number of private hospitals decreased by approximately 60% during this decade. The number of private hospitals beds also decreased by approximately 40% during the same period. In 1980 the private health sector represented 41.7% of total hospital beds, a percentage that decreased to 29.2% in 1995. The number of patients discharged from private for-profit hospitals decreased by 28% during the same period, representing only 19.3% of total hospital discharges in 1995.[17]

In the year 2004, as indicated by the data of the Ministry of Health & Social Solidarity, 196 private clinics were functioning in Greece with a total bed capacity of 15,260 in patient care beds (table 1).[18]

Table 1: Development of Private for profit health sector, Greece 1980 - 2004

		1980	1985	1990	1995	2000	2004
Number of Hospitals by legal status	Public	112	127	140	139	140	N/A
	LePL	28	15	3	4	5	N/A
	Private	468	318	244	215	192	196
Number of Hospital Beds by legal status	Public	25.905	32.646	35.896	36.717	35.730	N/A
	LePL	8.347	3.300	153	269	629	N/A
	Private	25.075	17.767	15.214	15.241	15.141	15.260
	Communal Health Centers	740	725	66	-	-	-
Number of Hospital beds by legal status, % total beds	Public	44.4%	61.3%	70.1%	70.3%	69.4%	N/A
	LePL	13.9%	6.1%	0.3%	0.5%	1.2%	N/A
	Private	41.7%	32.6%	29.6%	29.2%	29.4%	N/A
Patient discharged by hospital's legal status, % total patient discharged	Public	48.0%	67.0%	80,8%	80.2%	80.0%	N/A
	LePL	15.9%	8.1%	0.0%	0.5%	0.5%	N/A
	Private	35.9%	24.8%	19.2%	19.3%	19.5%	N/A
	Communal Health Centers	0.2%	0.1%	-	-	-	-

N/A: Not Available
LePL: Legal entity of Private Law
Sources: a. National Statistical Service of Greece. 1981 – 2003
b. National Statistical Service of Greece. 1981 – 2000
c. Ministry of Health & Social Solidarity. 2004

3. The post – NHS development period

The post – NHS development period of private for-profit health sector is characterised by three main features:

■ the high investment rate of private enterprises in biomedical technology

■ the selective focus of private enterprises on the development of the most profitable health care sectors

■ the absence of state control on the quality, the quantity and the type of health care services provided by the PFP health sector.

3.1 PFP health sector in Greece and biomedical technology: the case of Private Diagnostic Centers

The NHS foundation act (L.1397/83) as already mentioned prohibited the creation of new private hospitals and the expansion of those already functioning. Nevertheless the same law did not prohibit the setting up of private diagnostic centers. Since 1934 the state has allowed both medical doctors as well as private enterprises to set up microbiological and biological laboratories. These laboratories could exist either as separate enterprises or as departments within private clinics.[19]

The restrictive policy followed in the development of private clinics coexisted with concrete incentives to the private for-profit health sector to change its investment aims. PFP health sector took advantage of:

(a) the legislative oversight that allowed the foundation of private diagnostic centers;

(b) the fact that enterprises could easily, rapidly and without investing great amounts of money, acquire and renew their biomedical equipment through leasing;[20]

(c) the imposed inability of the public health sector to supply its hospitals with the necessary biomedical equipment, due to

Table 2: Private Diagnostic Centers, Greece 1980 – 2002

Year	Number of Private Diagnostic Centers
1980	12
1985	33
1991	192
1994	421
1996	403
2002	401

Sources: a. Besis N. 1993
b. ICAP. 1995-1997
c. Ministry of Health & Welfare. 2002

bureaucratic and finance problems

(d) the contracting policy with public sickness funds which offered a guaranteed income to the sector's enterprises

(e) the lack of an organized public Primary Health Care.

Taking advantage of all the above mentioned factors, in other words grasping the opportunity given by the state, the PFP health sector gave its attention to the development of outpatient care and diagnostic technology.

During the five year period from 1985 to 1991 private diagnostic centers (PDCs) rose by 582%, having a Median Annual Increase Rate of 25.8%.[20] During the next 3 years the number of PDC was over doubled.[21] And finally during the period from 1994 to 2002 the number of PDCs was stabilised (table 2).[22,23, b]

Another proof of the PFP health sector's growing investment in the area of biomedical technology stems from the time trend study of the ownership of high technology biomedical equipment (such as Computed Tomography Scanners, Magnetic Resonance Imaging Units, Lithotripts etc).

Although there is no official systematic data base of medical equipment installed both in public and private hospitals (including the medical equipment installed in PFP diagnostic centers) after having selected, elaborated and double checked five different sources and six different data bases[7,20,24,25,26,27] we are able to show that in 1985 PFP health sector possessed only the 33.3% of total CT Scanners all over the country. Since then, PFP health enterprises (included PDC) have become dominant in the area of high technology medical equipment, and by 2002 they possessed 67.9% of total CT scanners and 80% of total MRI units (table 3).

The per capita ratio of this type of medical equipment in Greece out-

Table 3: Biomedical Technology in Public and Private Health Sector, Greece 1980 - 2002

		1980	1985	1990	1992	1997	2002
Number of Computed Tomography Scanners	Public	4	10	22	22	41	75
	Private	2	5	44	99	104	159
Number of Magnetic Resonance Imaging Units	Public	0	N/A	2	2	N/A	19
	Private	1	N/A	2	7	N/A	76

N/A: Not Available
Public: included National Health System, Hospitals LePL, Military Hospitals
Private: included Private Clinics, Private Diagnostic Centers

Sources: a. Besis N. 1993
       b. Kyriopoulos G. Niakas D. 1994
       c. ICAP. 2001 – 2003
       d. OECD. 2004
       e. Ministry of Health & Welfare. 2003

strips the average per capita ratio among the countries of the European Union (in 2002 the ratio of CT scanners and MRI units per million population in Greece was 21.34 and 8.7 respectively while in EU-15 countries the corresponding figures were 16.87 and 7.04).[7,27] This is the outcome of the investment activity of PFP enterprises. Medical equipment provision in Greece, at least as far as the private health sector is concerned, has never been under any state control. Many researchers therefore believe that the increased rate of the provision and diffusion of hi-tech biomedical equipment, caused by private health enterprises, is related in one way or another to induced supplier demand for unnecessary medical examinations.[20,28]

It is generally asserted, but not proved, that 70 – 90% of private diagnostic centers' revenue is obtained from public sickness funds.[26,3] The lack of necessary technological equipment in public hospitals leads patients to 'consume' medical services from the private health sector, causing the economic 'bleeding' of public sickness funds.[28,29] As it can be seen in 1998 IKA's (IKA: Institute of Social Insurance, is the largest sickness fund in Greece having in the year 2001 more than 5.5 million blue and white collar workers and their dependents as directly or indirectly insured members) [30] payments for medical examinations held in PFP Diagnostic Centers were more than EUR 35 million (table 4).[31]

3.2 The selective development of private enterprises on the most profitable health care sectors in Greece

As already mentioned, in the post-NHS era the PFP health enterprises have focused selectively only on the profitable health care sectors.

It is generally accepted that PFP health sector is developed by meeting the demand and not the need for health care services.[32] In other words the private sector lacks in community benefit: for example the for-profit hospitals do not produce their share of public goods, such as charity care, medical education and research.[33]

This allegation seems to stand in the case of the Greek Private Health

Table 4: IKA's payments for medical examinations held in Private for – profit Diagnostics Centers, Greece 1998

	Number of Patients	Payments
Athens	219.817	10.855.476 €
Province	363.823	24.973.666 €
Total	583.640	35.829.143 €
Source: Fyntanidou E. 2000		

Sector. During the post-NHS period private sector, confirming the inverse care law ("the availability of good medical care tends to vary inversely with the need of it in the population served. This inverse care law operates more completely where medical care is most exposed to market forces"),[34] did not regionalise its services. On the opposite it gathered them even more in the urban areas where higher demand for medical care is taken for granted.

As it can be seen, in 1980 the private sector had already gathered 70% of its inpatient care beds in the districts of Athens and Thessaloniki.[16] Since then the accumulation of private inpatient care beds in urban centers has grown even larger (table 5). In 2002 – 2004 PFP sector concentrated 80% of its inpatient care beds[18] and 75% of its diagnostic laboratories[23] in the districts of Athens and Thessaloniki.

Similar conclusions can be reached by the study of the distribution of private in-patient care beds by specialty. One can ascertain that private enterprises have high penetration rates in the areas of Obstetrics-Gynaecology, Neuro-Psychiatry, Nephrology and Otorhinolaryngology in patient care beds, and low penetration rates in areas such as Neonatology, Coronary and Oncology and Radiotherapeutic Units (table 6).[17] One can also ascertain that although the private sector is dominant in the area of Obstetric and Gynecology Clinics it possesses only a small number of Neonatology Units, a fact that causes a constant patient flow from Private Clinics to Public Hospitals.

Finally, the selective development of private heath sector can easily be shown from a study of movement by legal status and specialty of hospitals. In 1995, approximately 85% of Obstetric – Gynaecology and 37.4% of Neuropsychiatry patients were discharged from private clinics. In the same period (1996) approximately 30% of surgical operations were carried out in private clinics.[17]

Table 5: Private for profit Hospital Beds by geographic region, % total PFP hospital beds, Greece 1980 – 2004

Geographic Region	1980	1985	1990	1995	2000	2004
Greater Athens	47.4	49.8	52.6	53.2	51.9	56.4
Rest of Central Greece & Evia	5.1	4.5	3.7	4.0	3.5	2.6
Peloponnissos	4.9	3.9	3.5	2.9	2.6	1.9
Ionian Islands	0.5	0.6	0.5	0.4	0.4	0.3
Ipiros	1.5	1.4	1.0	0.6	0.3	0.2
Thessalia	8.2	9.0	9.2	10.1	11.1	11.0
Macedonia (Thessaloniki)	23.3	24.7	24.2	23.5	25.5	24.2
Thraki	2.0	0.9	0.6	0.6	0.4	0.4
Aegean Islands	1.2	0.9	0.9	0.7	0.7	0.7
Kriti	5.8	4.3	3.8	4.1	3.7	2.3
Sources: a. National Statistical Service of Greece. 1981 – 2003 b. Ministry of Health & Social Solidarity. 2004						

3.3 The absence of state control on health care services provided by the PFP health sector in Greece

As already mentioned, one of the main characteristics of the development of the private sector during the post-NHS period is the absence of governmental control on the quality, quantity and type of health care services that it delivers.

At this point it is necessary to mention that since 1925 the law (the act of 18/10/1925) has allowed private enterprises to run Infectious Diseases and Tubercular Hospitals.[35] Three legislative frameworks followed, which determined the conditions, the prerequisites and the specification frames of operation of private clinics in Greece.[36] Between 1962-1963 the Royal Acts (451/62 and 521/63) were to set, for the first time, technical and constructional specifications for the operation of private clinics and the required number of nursing and medical staff.[37,38] In 1983 the foundation act of NHS forbade the founding, the take-over or the displacement of private hospitals.[3] In 1991 the conservative government of the New Democracy Party decided – enforcing Presidential Act 247/91 – on the liberalisation of the health care market, suspending article 6 of the foundation act of NHS, allowing in this way the establishment of new private hospitals.[39] Also, during the same period, the New Democracy government updated the private clinics' operational requirements, making them stricter[40], with the Presidential Act 517/91.

The transition to a new government in 1993 and the assumption of power by the social democrats did not bring any change in the legislative framework of private clinics, despite the fact that prior to the elections the social democrat party had promised to abolish acts 517 and 247 of 1991. In 2000 the social democrats updated the operational framework of those private clinics that had acquired operating licences through 1962-63 Royal Acts, by passing

Table 6: Private for profit hospital beds by specialty of clinics, % total (public and private) hospital beds by specialty, Greece 1996

PFP Hospital Beds by specialty	% total
All specialties	29.07%
Obstetrics - Gynaecology	52.81%
Neuro - Psychiatry	38.31%
Otorhinolaryngology	33.47%
Nephrology	29.73%
Surgical	28.83%
Pathology	23.69%
Neonatology	12.54%
Paediatrics	8.73%
Coronary Units	6.33%
Oncology – Chemotherapy, Radiotherapeutic	5.04%

Source: National Statistical Service of Greece. 2000

Table 7: Legislation on Private for profit clinics, Greece

Legislation	Number of clinics (% total clinics)	
	2002	2004
Royal Decrees 451/62, 521/63	186 (94.9%)	56 (28.9%)
Presidential Decrees 247/91, 517/91	10 (5.1%)	11 (5.7%)
Presidential Decree 235/00	-	127 (65.5%)
Source: Ministry of Health and Social Solidarity. 2004		

the Presidential act 235/2000.[41]

According to data provided by the Ministry of Health and Social Welfare, in 2002 95% of private clinics were operating according to the Royal Acts of 1962-1963 and only 5% were operating under the legislation of 1991 (table 7).[18]

What happened in 1990s was that the clinic proprietors after the enforcement of 517/91 moved towards taking over old clinics that were operating under the Royal Acts of 1962-1963.[42] Practically this meant that 11 years after the liberalization of health market by the conservatives, the private health sector continued to operate without any governmental control and with operational conditions and requirements of the 1960s.

4. Contemporary development characteristics of PFP Health Sector in Greece

Today the private health sector in Greece is growing rapidly, a growth which is characterized by :

(a) the high rate of revenue increase

(b) an increase in the number of mergers and acquisitions, which progressively led to the development of oligopolistic enterprises in the Greek of private for-profit health market

(c) the entry of insurance firms to the health care sector and the verticalisation of their services according to HMO patterns.

According to market estimates the Median Annual Increase Rate of revenues in the private health sector between 1993-2002 reached 12.9% (table 8).[21,22,25,26] In 2002 the revenues of the private sector reached 1 billion euro.

Two basic reasons leading to the take over of small enterprises by bigger ones are the difficulty of the small units of the sector

(a) to respond to the exponential growth of medical technology, and

(b) the high construction cost of a new therapeutic unit according to the current framework.

This merger and acquisition procedure is reflected, up to a degree, in the increased median bed capacity of private clinics in Greece which in 1980 was 53.6 beds per clinic, while in 2002 it was 78 beds per clinic.[16]

Today corporate groups are operating in the health sector, many of which have already signed contracts with private health insurance companies offering a complete spectrum of medical and diagnostic services (inpatient care, diagnostic tests, ambulatory care). An indication of the development of oligopolistic enterprises in the health sector is the fact that 8 enterprises absorb 70.2% of the total revenues of general hospitals' sector, 3 enterprises absorb 79% of the total revenues of obstetrics hospitals sector, and finally 12 enterprises absorb 45.4% of the diagnostic centres' turnover.[26]

5. Conclusion

In Greece until the early 1980s private for profit health sector was dominant. The foundation of the National Health System in 1983 had a great impact on the PFP sector. During the period 1985 to 1995 private hospitals decreased by 60%, private bed clinics decreased by 40% and patient discharged from private clinics decreased by 28%.

In the post-NHS era, three are the main development characteristics of PFP health sector:

● the high investment rates in biomedical technology causing, in a very short period, the dominance of private enterprises in the area of high technology biomedical equipment, a fact that is strongly related both to induced supplier demand for unnecessary medical tests as well as to the economic 'bleeding' of public sickness funds

● the selective development of private enterprises in the most prof-

Table 8: Revenues of Private for Profit Health Sector, Greece 1993 – 2002

	General & NeuroPsychiatry Clinics	Obstetrics - Gynaecology Clinics	Diagnostic Centers
1993	219.22		97.72
1994	246.51		108.58
1995	219.84	45.48	121.49
1996	247.98	58.69	135.28
1997	265.60	88.60	153.80
1998	293.50	110.30	170.20
1999	343.70	120.90	183.10
2000	395.00	140.60	203.10
2001	455.80	150.00	227.70
2002	539.30	164.00	241.00
All amounts in million €. Private medical consultants revenues not included			
Sources: ICAP, 1995 – 2003			

itable health care sectors, causing both the accumulation of private for profit inpatient care beds in the districts of Athens and Thessaloniki as well as the high penetration rates of private enterprises in the sectors of Obstetrics, Neuro Psychiatry, Nephrology and Surgery Clinics

● the absence of governmental control, causing, until the year 2002, the operation of private clinics under the technical and constructural specification frames set by the Royal Acts, enforced in the early 1960s.

Today in Greece, through a process of hospital mergers and acquisition, oligopolistic corporate groups operate in the private health care industry, creating vertically or virtually integrated health systems by contacting with private health insurance companies and by offering a complete spectrum of diagnostic and medical services.

This analysis of the development characteristics of the PFP health providers indicates that private sector in Greece was literally sponsored by the governments' policies. The legislative oversight and facilitation, the absence of state control on the type, quantity and quality of health care services provided by the private sector, the contracting policy of public sickness funds which offers a guaranteed income to the sector's enterprises, indicate the attachment of both social-democratic and conservative governments to the ensuring and promoting of corporate interests in the health care sector in Greece.

Additionally, the policies of underfunding the public sector, the fragmentation of social insurance and public health services, the lack of an organized public primary health care, policies of understaffing (especially with nurses), the informal payments and the shortage of medical equipment and accommodation in public hospitals (aspects not thoroughly discussed in this paper, as they exceed the scope and limits of our analysis) created an environment of imposed failings and dissatisfaction for the public health sector, leading to an increased demand for private health services.

Our analysis shows that privatisation of health care in Greece was and still is a deliberate policy choice rather than a spontaneous reaction of the private health industry to the 'inborn inabilities' of the public health sector.

Notes

a Privatisation is described as the process in which non-government actors become increasingly involved in the financing and provision of health care services[9]

b In this point it is of great importance to mention that there is no official record of PDC operating around the country. The evidence we present is the outcome of the selection and processing of 3 different sources and 4 different data bases.

C Most sickness funds in Greece are Legal Entities of Private Law. Some of them are wholly funded by the state (such as Organization of Agricultural Insurance – OFA) and others receive state subsidies (such as the Institute of Social Insurance – IKA).

References

1 Kyriopoulos G, Niakas D. Health care financing in Greece. Center of Health Social Sciences. Athens. 1991:41-50 [in Greek]

2 General Secretariat of Social Insurance. Social Budget Years 2002. Ministry of Labour and Social Insurance. Athens 2002:345-430

3 OECD. *Private health insurance in OECD countries*. Organisation for Economic Co-operation and Development. Paris. 2004

4 Tsalikis G. Foundation of (anti)social insurance in Greece (1840-1940). In: Kyriopoulos G, Liaropoulos L, Boursanidis C, Economou C. *Social insurance in Greece*. Themelio. Athens. 2001:19-47 [in Greek]

5 Venieris D. Health policy in Greece: the history of reform. In: Kyriopoulos G, Sissouras A. *Unified Sickness Fund: necessity and illusion*. Themelio. Athens 1997:151-72 [in Greek]

6 WHO. National Health Accounts. World Health Organization 2004 (Cited April, 2005): www.who.int/nha/country/GRC.xls

7 OECD. Health Data. *A comparative analysis of 30 countries*. 3rd edition (CD ROM). Organisation for Economic Co-operation and Development. Paris. 2004

8 Navarro V. ed. *The political economy of social inequalities. Consequences for health and quality of life*. Baywood. New York. 2002

9 Kumaranayake L. *Effective regulation of private sector health service providers*. The World Bank 1998 (Cited April, 2005): www.worldbank.org/wbi/mdf/mdf2/papers/humandev/health/kumaranayake

10 Antonopoulou A. Le système de santé en Grèce et son intégration dans l'environnement économique et social (Thèse pour la doctorat 3éme cycle «Economie de ressources humaines» mention «économie de la santé»). Université de Dijon. 1979

11 Law 1397. National Health System. Government's Newspaper A' no 143. Athens. 7/10/1983

12 Polyzos N. Secondary, Tertiary Care. In: Ministry of Health and Welfare ed. *Study for the designing and organization of health care system*. Athens. 1994:147-58 [in Greek]

13 Kyriopoulos G, Georgousi E, Drizi M. Investment in biotechnology in Greece. In: Kyriopoulos G, Levet G, Niakas D. ed. *Management of biotechnology in Greece*. Center of Health Social Sciences. Athens. 1994:145-54 [in Greek]

14 Yfantopoulos G. *Planning of health sector in Greece. Economic and social dimensions*. National Center of Social Studies. Athens. 1988:85-94 [in Greek]

15 Matsaganis M. From the North Sea to the Mediterranean? Constraints to health reform in Greece. *Int J Health Serv* 1998;28:333-48

16 National Statistical Service of Greece. *Statistical Yearbook of Greece*. Athens. 1981 - 2003

17 National Statistical Service of Greece. *Social Welfare and Health Statistics 1980 - 1996*. Athens. 1981-2000

18 Ministry of Health & Social Solidarity. Department of private clinics. Athens. 8/10/2004

19 Presidential Decree. Institution and inspection of Microbiological and Biological Diagnostic Laboratories. Government's Newspaper A' no 384. Athens. 3/11/1934

20 Besis N. *Private health services. The sectors of private diagnostic centers, private clinics and rehabilitation centers*. Institute of Economic and Industrial Studies. Athens. 1993 [in Greek]

21 ICAP. Private Health Services. ICAP AE. Athens. 1995

22 ICAP. Private Health Services. ICAP AE. Athens. 1997

23 Ministry of Health and Welfare. Health Map. Athens. 2002 (Cited July, 2003): www.healthgis.ariadne-t.gr/healthmap/

24 Kyriopoulos G, Niakas D. *Issues of Economics and Health Policy*. Center of Social Health Studies. Athens. 1994 [in Greek]

25 ICAP. Private Health Services. ICAP AE. Athens. 2001

26 ICAP. Private Health Services. ICAP AE. Athens. 2003

27 Ministry of Health & Welfare. *Study of high technology equipment installation in NHS hospitals*. EKEVYL AE. Athens. 2003

28 Theodorou M, Sarris M, Soulis S. *Health systems*. Papazisis. Athens. 2001:210, 273-4, 280-1 [in Greek]

29 Karokis A. Sissouras A. Organization and financing. In: Ministry of Health and Welfare ed. *Study for the designing and organization of health care system*. Athens. 1994:57-8 [in Greek]

National health policy and the ongoing reforms in the field of occupational health in the Republic of Macedonia

J.Karadzinska -Bislimovska, S.Risteska-Kuc

Introduction

A process of economical and political transition has been underway in Republic of Macedonia ever since independence in 1991, with reform in all sectors, including the health care system. In the framework of relevant systematic changes in national health policy, planned reform activities in the field of occupational health should provide the main goals: the protection and promotion of health of working people. Socio-economic conditions, the introduction of the market economy, high rate of unemployment as well as previous political and war crisis have all had a negative impact on the health and safety issue in the country.

The recognized problems in this area – old and new specific occupational risks, inadequate function of occupational health services and labour inspection services, and the insufficiency of the occupational health information system – require fundamental changes in the principles of managing occupational health and safety, the establishment of modern occupational health services and introduction of new mechanisms for social dialogue as vision for the future.

New reform concept

New reform concepts in occupational health and safety sector in the country are based on the adaptation of the policy, system and services to the new political and socio-economic conditions according to the requirements of international criteria (WHO, ILO, EU).

A common and important starting point of the reforms is that ever since 1950s the occupational health system has been an integral part of the general health care system in Republic of Macedonia. Specific occupational health activities are conducted through a network of occupational health units, mostly in Health Centres at municipal level, fewer at enterprise level, provided by the highly educated and qualified staff of 200 professionals including 120 occupational health specialists.

The reduced number of OH units, which carry out specific OH activities, characterizes the current situation and there is also an evident transformation of OH specialists to GP or family doctors, all in the frame of ongoing health care reforms.

The Institute of Occupational Health – the WHO Collaborating Centre for Occupational Health – plays an important and leading role in educational, scientific and specific health care issues in occupational health in the Republic of Macedonia.

The Institute as a member of the Global Network of WHO Collaborating Centers in Occupational Health provides a realisation of specific WHO program activities at national and international level. Evidence for this is the involvement of the country as a member of the Executive team in the current WHO European Programme "Health in the World of Work" national occupational health policies, and services in transition economies module.

It also has a leading role in ongoing reforms in the occupational health sector. The Institute of Occupational Health, supported by the Macedonian Society of Occupational Health, should have the main role in implementation of occupational health reform activities in addition to the positive reform political orientation in the country in this domain.

Taking all this into consideration, now is the crucial moment to emphasize the need for organization and the establishment of an adequate new model of OHS and to establish new rules in occupational health system and policy in Republic of Macedonia.

It is very important that this issue is officially supported by the

"Occupational health and safety at work "priority in the Biennial Collaborative Agreement between the Ministry of Health in Macedonia and the WHO Regional Office for Europe which is proceeding in the next period.

Key elements for action

In particular, the adequate role and function of OHS is to be defined through legislative tools and basis, professional human resources and objectives of the national strategy for Health, Healthy Environment and Safety at Work, directed by Ministry of Health.

In April 2005 the most important event was the National Conference of Health and Safety at work, supported by WHO Regional Office for Europe and Ministry of Health, with an intersectoral and multidisciplinary profile and participation of occupational health experts from South East European countries. The conclusions and recommendations springing out from it, specifically the National Strategy for Health, Healthy Environment and Safety at Work and the proposed model for occupational health services are in line with WHO recommendations.

Legislative tools such as the Labour and Work Protection Code, Health protection Code, Environment protection Code, as well as adopted WHO and ILO documents (ILO Conventions and WHO Strategy on Occupational Health for All) are a solid basis for reforms and future development in this sector.

The adoption and implementation by the Government of National strategy for Health, Healthy Environment and Safety at Work should give support to a national framework and should promote intersectoral collaboration of different stakeholders (occupational health professionals, ministries and authorities, inspections, science and education, employers' and employees' associations, NGOs etc) in the field of occupational health and safety.

According to the National Strategy an Intersectoral Committee has to be established at Governmental level, and this would help the implementation of the national occupational health and safety strategy based on common goals through social dialogue.

The basic principles of the Strategy refer to:

■ primary prevention and safe technology,

■ innovation and harmonisation to the legislation and standards in the area,

■ optimisation of work conditions,

■ integration of all measures and activities,

■ a tripartite approach (Government, Employers, Employees),

■ cooperation of employers and employees,

■ the right of the employees to adequate information and participation in decision making concerning occupational health,

■ surveillance and promotion of health, safety and protection systems as well as development of registration and data systems.

The principles support the WHO concept of good practice of health, healthy living and working environment and safety management in enterprises (Health, Environment and Safety Management in Enterprises – HESME) promoted in Republic of Macedonia in 2001. This increases the responsibility of the Government for establishing health protection and health promotion of the population as a priority. It also gives direction to the activities that should be implemented through national legislation according to the available means and capacities of the country as well as regional and international cooperation.

The multidisciplinary approach is a very strong impulse to occupational health reforms, which has created applicable instruments for allocation of occupational health problems.

Updating national legislation in occupational health and safety and the establishment of a new model of occupational health services within the public OHS network on national, local and enterprise level are priorities of the National Strategy.

To strengthen basic occupational health services, to expand their coverage and to improve their content and activities are the key points of the reform process.

The sub regional approach is a new perspective in the development of Occupational Health policy, system and services in the country. This is initiated by WHO CCs meeting in Stockholm, September 2003, focused as a WHO-ILO Project proposal "Strengthening social dialogue for improving occupational health and safety in South East Europe".

In the framework of the National Conference of Health and Safety at work a Sub-regional Consultation was held on Developing Projects for Occupational Health for South East Europe, under the Initiative for Social Cohesion of the Stability Pact.

The project on strengthening social dialogue for improving occupational health and safety in South East Europe encompasses the idea that occupational health and safety are recognized by the health and labour sector as an area for partnership, collaboration and joint action.

This project is a very important step forward to ongoing changes in the field of occupational health and safety.

Conclusion

Elaboration and implementation of the new key elements in occupational health and safety and supporting the initiation of a regional approach for social cohesion in the field of the workplace health policy is a challenge for national health policy and the ongoing reforms in the field of occupational health in Republic of Macedonia. It is also a challenge for the new view in the public health strategy in Europe.

References:

1. National Strategy for Health, Healthy Environment and Safety at Work, Ministry of Health, Republic of Macedonia, 2005 (in procedure)
2. Karadzinska-Bislimovska J, Baranski B, Risteska-Kuc S. Health, environment and social management in enterprises programme in Republic of Macedonia.Med Lav 2004; (95),1:55-61

Health care policy in Palestine: challenges and opportunities

Motasem Hamdan, PhD

1. Background

Since the Oslo Peace agreement in 1993, the Palestinian health system context is characterized by political and economic destabilization (Hamdan & Defever, 2002). The authority over the Palestinian health care system was transferred to the Palestinian in 1994. Previously a division of the Israeli Ministry of Defence administered the public clinics and hospitals.

Since the changeover, fundamental changes in the system have taken place; the most discernible of these have been in the governmental health services. Reforms included expanding and enhancing health care provision capacity, improving the management, developing of human resources, and adjusting of public financing and health insurance scheme. The aim of these reform initiatives was to reconstruct the system and to assure the provision of appropriate services for the entire Palestinian population. These issues will be tackled later in this analysis (Hamdan, 2003).

Palestinian health care is characterised by heterogeneity and fragmentation of public and private provision and funding arrangements (Hamdan et. al, 2003). Health is care provided by four major mechanisms;

● the public sector, represented mainly by the Ministry of Health (MoH),

● United Nation Relief and Working Agency in Near East (UNRWA),

● non-governmental organisations (NGOs),

● and a private for-profit health sector.

Health care is financed by a mixture of resources, the main source is private out of pocket spending, then public spending through taxation and revenues of the Governmental Health Insurance (GHI) scheme, third international sources, and finally by non-governmental sources.

This analysis focuses on the recent policy changes with regard to financing and providing health care in Palestine and especially those concerning the role of private health sector and its impact on the availability and accessibility to health care.

2. Financing and insurance

Major policy trends concerning health care financing after the changeover can be summarized in three areas. The first was increasing public/governmental contributions to financing health care services. This has been evident from the development in the budget of the MoH. Governmental spending on healthcare increased from US$ 62million in 1994 to US$ 134 million in 2004 (MoH, 2005) (Fig.1).

The second was shift in the sources of public spending with reliance on general tax revenues instead of the revenues of the GHI; for example the percentage of GHI revenues decreased from 19% in 1991 to only 8% in 1997 (World Bank, 1998).

The third major policy change with regard to financing has been expanding the coverage of the GHI scheme, through opening the scheme for voluntary enrolment by those who were not required to participate, reducing premiums, and providing free insurance coverage for

Sources of data: (MoH, 2003;2004;2005)

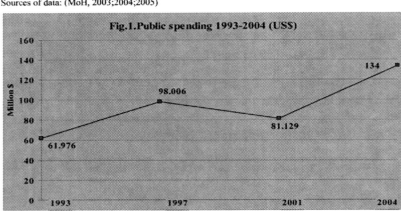

Fig.1.Public spending 1993-2004 (US$)

vulnerable families after the eruption of the Palestinian Intifada in November 2000.

This public policy has impacted positively on the number of households enrolled in the public insurance scheme (Fig.2). While in 1993 only 20% of the Palestinian families was covered by this scheme, the number reached 55% of the families in 2004 and 29.5% of these families were insured free of charge (MoH,2005).

3. Provision of health care

In the provision of health care there has been a consistent public policy toward improving the availability and accessibility to health care through:

3.1. Strengthening the public sector capacity in the health care delivery

In the public health sector, the number of governmental health facilities increased significantly after 1994 (Fig.3, Fig.4). For example the number of governmental PHC clinics increased from 205 in 1994 to 391 clinics in 2003 – an increase of 91%, and the public hospital beds increased from 1852 in 1994 to reach 2735 in 2004 – an increase of 47% (MoH, 2005).

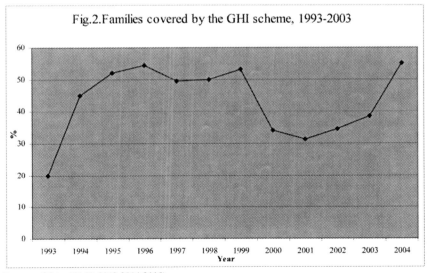

Fig.2.Families covered by the GHI scheme, 1993-2003

Sources of data: (MoH, 2003;2004;2005)

3.2. Promoting the private health sector (both for-profit and non-for-profit NGO) role in health care delivery

An important sector in providing health care in Palestine is the private health sector. It includes all those working outside the direct state control both for and not-for profit practices e.g. NGOs. But within this sector our focus is on the private for-profit practices, that accessibility to

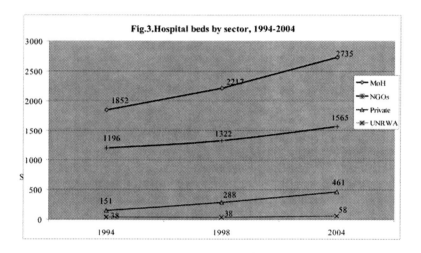

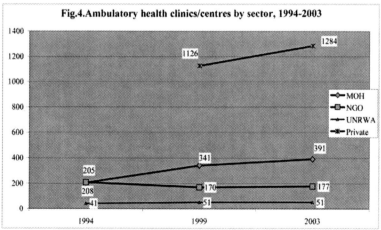

MoH, NGOs and UNRWA's sector consists of PHC clinics of different levels.
Private for-profit sector consists of self-employed GP, specialists physicians and dental clinics
Source of data (MoH, 2003;2004)

be determined by the ability and willingness of the people to pay for services.

The general characteristics of the private for-profit health sector in Palestine (which is similar to those in other countries) that it has an important role in providing ambulatory medical care services, and mainly focuses on curative medical care. Moreover, private practices are prevalent where the well-off population is concentrated for example in Palestine in the urban areas, and in the West Bank more than in the Gaza Strip, for economic reasons. And, it has significantly grown after 1994 with the prospects of peace and stability after the Oslo Peace Agreement.

Fig.4 shows that the private for-profit health practices constitute an important source for ambulatory health care services in comparison with other sectors. Although adequate information about private for-profit practices is missing, based on the available data this figure provides a comparable data about ambulatory care clinics and centres in Palestine and their recent growth in comparison with services provided by other sectors between 1999 and 2003. Yet, it is important to indicate that those facilities owned by the Ministry of Health, UNRWA and NGOs are PHC clinics and centres from different levels, and those owned by the private for profit sector consists of the practices of self employed dentists and GPs as well as specialised physicians.

Fig.5 shows more detailed data about the types of services mainly

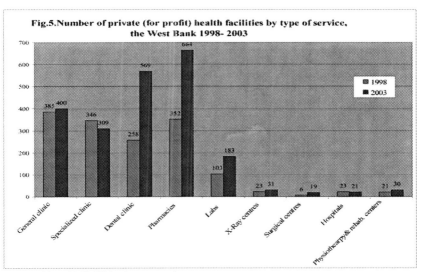

Fig.5.Number of private (for profit) health facilities by type of service, the West Bank 1998- 2003

Sources of data (MoH, 2005, private contact)

provided by the private for-profit sector in the West Bank, where the private practices are more prevalent than in Gaza Strip. These services are: dental clinics, GP and specialist practices, pharmacies, medical laboratories, radiology and imaging centres, physiotherapy clinics, and maternity and obstetrics hospitals.

The figure also shows the recent considerable growth in the number of these practices between 1998 and 2003, where the most important increases have been in the number of dental clinics and private pharmacies, which were doubled over the same period (Fig.5). This increase is due to graduation of many pharmacist and dentists from local universities which started these programmes after 1994.

But, if we look at the role of for-profit private sector in provision of hospital care (Fig.6), we can see that similar to public and non-governmental sectors, there has been a significant increase in the number of for-profit beds since 1994. For example the total number of private beds in 1998 was twice the 1994 level, and in 2003 it was more than three times the 1994 level (MoH, 2004).

Private for-profit beds form a small percentage of the total available beds in Palestine, only about 11% in 2003. It worth mentioning that 13 out of the available 21 private hospitals in the West Bank are very small maternity and obstetrics hospitals (about 47% of the private beds in Palestine (MoH, 2004)). This is due to the significant demand for these services as a result of the high fertility rates among Palestinians and due to the shortness of length of stay at these hospitals.

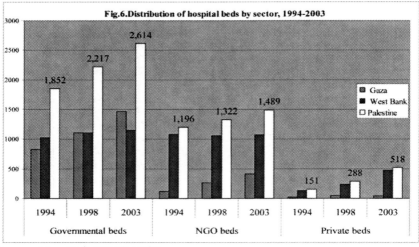

Sources of data: (MoH, 2003;2004;2005)

4. Reasons behind the growth of the private sector

Given the considerable growth of the private for-profit health care supply that has been witnessed lately, it seems evident that there has been a public policy trend towards promoting private health care provision based on the conviction that the private sector can positively contribute to the provision of health care services. Many factors have affected the growth of the sector. There is a lack of proper regulating processes of the private sector, particularly the accreditation and licensing of private facilities is very weak.

Another important reason is the shortages of the public sector capacity in provision and quality of health care. The MoH is contracting out tertiary health care to private providers: its services are generally perceived as low quality and there are geographic imbalances in the distribution of public services. However, we believe that there are other factors which have also played an important role in the increase in private sector such as the prospects of political stability and economic security in the post-Oslo period, and finally, the donor driven policies and their influence towards promoting the private health sector and decreasing state involvement in health care provision.

5. Impact of private for-profit health sector on the availability and on the accessibility to health care services

In order to determine the impact of private for-profit health sector on the availability and on the accessibility to health care services, first we need to look at the types of health services provided by the private for-profit sector and then examine accessibility to these services by different population groups.

Fig.7 presents the numbers and types of the licensed private for-profit practices by regions. Based on these and earlier comparable figures two main conclusions can be made. First, there are many services that are considerably made available by the private for-profit sector and can be summarized as follows:

● Specialized medical services

● Day care surgery services

● Hi-tech radiology and imaging services

● Specialized dental care services

- Advanced medical laboratories
- Hospital care, basically maternity and obstetrics services.

However, these services are less prevalent in Gaza than in West Bank, where the socio-economic conditions are better. And even in the West Bank, these services are mainly available in urban areas, lesser in rural and almost not available in the refugee camps where poverty is widespread.

As for the impact of the private for-profit practices on the accessibility to health services, we say in principle the accessibility to private for-profit services is determined by the ability and willingness to pay. Given that currently about 65% of the population are living below the poverty line, which means less than US$ 2 per day (World Bank, 2004), – and also due to the fact that private for profit services are not cheap – we can conclude that the accessibility is very limited.

But, there is another important factor in determining the accessibility to private for-profit practices: that is health insurance. Therefore in order to examine the accessibility of private for profit services it necessary also to look at the available health insurance schemes and their coverage packages. In Palestine people can be divided into four groups according to health insurance coverage (PCBS, 2004; MoH, 2004):

Those covered by the GHI, about 55% of the Palestinian households. But this insurance covers only public providers unless the patient is referred to the private sector for care not available by the MoH. Most of these cases are limited to tertiary care.

Registered refugees, about 33% of the households, covered by

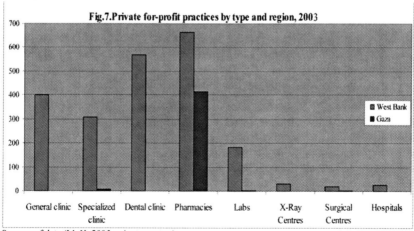

Fig.7.Private for-profit practices by type and region, 2003

Sources of data (MoH, 2005, private contact)

UNRWA health system services. UNRWA also mainly covers services available at its clinics, yet it subcontracts limited services to private providers, but patients have to contribute significantly to the cost of services.

Those enrolled in private insurance schemes, about 8% of the households. Private insurance schemes cover specific service packages provided by different health sectors including the private health sector.

And lastly, those without any health insurance coverage, among them the well off who prefer to purchase their own health services and the low risk population e.g. young people preferring out-of-pocket payment.

In conclusion, given the available insurance schemes in Palestine and their coverage we can say that the utilisation of private for-profit services is largely dependent on out of pocket spending, and that creates inequity in accessibility between different socio-economic groups.

Conclusions

In Palestine, the weakness of the governmental capacity to provide health care and lack of proper regulating mechanisms, prospects of peace and stability as well donors influence have contributed to the flourishing of the private for-profit health sector since 1994.

Although policies of promoting the private health sector have had positive impact on the availability of medical health services, it has created inequitable patterns of accessibility between different socio-economic groups.

Therefore, policies ensuring adequate integration and complementarity, accompanied by appropriate monitoring and regulation by the government (the Ministry of Health) are necessary to improve the efficient use of limited resources, and improve the quality of care. They can at the same time offer choice alternatives to patients.

References

Four Years – Intifada, Closures and Palestinian Economic Crisis: an Assessment, the World Bank, 2004.

Hamdan M, Defever M, Abdeen Z. Organising Health Care within Political Turmoil: The Palestinian Case. *Int J Health Plann Manage* 2003;18(1):63-88.

Hamdan M, Defever M. A "transitional" context for health policy development: The Palestinian case. *Health Policy* 2002; 59(3):193-207.

Hamdan M. The dynamics of health policy development during transition and under uncertainty: what can be learned from the Palestinian experience?

Acta Hospitalia. Issue 3, 2003.

Health status in Palestine: annual report 2002. Ministry of Health, Gaza, Palestine, 2003.

Health status in Palestine: annual report 2003. Ministry of Health, Gaza, Palestine, 2004.

Health status in Palestine: annual report 2004. Ministry of Health, Gaza, Palestine, 2005.

Palestinian Central Bureau of Statistics (PCBS), 2003. Percentage of health insurance coverage 2000-3.

West Bank and Gaza: Medium-Term Development Strategy for the Health Sector. Washington DC: The World Bank, 1998.

Health care system in Serbia: Present state and reform

Prof. Slobodan Jankovic

The health care system in Serbia has not changed very much in the last 50 years. New laws on health care, health insurance and chambers of health workers were passed in the Parliament in December 2005[1,2,3,] but their effect remains to be seen. There are two sectors: a public health care system, funded, maintained, and controlled by the state; and a private health care system. The public health care system is funded through state-owned health insurance, contribution to which is obligatory for each citizen of Serbia with regular income. Each health care facility agrees a separate contract with the health insurance, through which it is funded. The private health sector is permitted to cover only primary health care. Private health care facilities can make contracts with state-owned health insurance, or may charge patients directly for their services.

Health care is guaranteed for each citizen, regardless of his (or her) social status. Unemployed, school children and students, persons older than 65 years of age, disabled and even minorities without permanent place of living are granted equal access to health care as employed persons who regularly contribute to the health insurance funds. However, there is a clause in the health care law which identifies that access to healthcare services is provided in accordance with financial situation of the health insurance system. In order to regulate access to expensive health interventions (e.g. expensive antineoplastic agents, organ transplantation, prosthetic implants, etc.) the state health insurance fund has developed an elaborate system of lists of allowable drugs and expert commissions, which operates centrally, through the four tertiary health care institutions, called Clinical centers, and located in the four major cities of Serbia (Belgrade, Nis, Novi Sad and Kragujevac). Since the cost of drugs is only reimbursed to patients after they have been prescribed and used by the patient, this system can lead to conflict.

The public health care system organizes primary, secondary and tertiary health care. Primary health care is organized through huge health care facilities called 'Dom Zdravlija', or "Home of Health", where patients come for the services of general practitioners and certain specialists (paediatricians and gynaecologists). Although the intention is that each patient can choose their primary care physician, because of the current organisation of "Homes of Health" it is not yet possible in majority of cases. Patients are obliged to attend the health care facilities, with home visits reserved only for patients confined to bed. It is not yet possible to make appointments with general practitioners, and the patients are obliged to keep their own medical records, since only limited data on previous visits to general practitioners are kept in the patients' files in "Homes of Health".

For urgent health problems citizens can refer directly to the "Urgent medical service", a separate department of "Home of Health". This service is also available on call, and will dispatch teams (composed of a physician and a nurse) to the medical emergency.

Secondary and tertiary health care is organized in hospitals, graded from general hospitals (secondary care only), through clinical-hospital centers (mixed secondary and tertiary care) to clinical centers (tertiary care) The hospitals are financed directly from the Health insurance fund (based on annual contracts), and are controlled directly from the Ministry of Health. The Republic of Serbia government appoints managers and management boards of the hospitals directly, on the basis of proposal made by the Minister of Health. This system of appointment has brought many problems in the functioning of the hospitals, because in the past it provided for direct influence of political parties on internal organization and expert work of the hospitals, and there has been a marked lack of continuity of management following each political reorganization.

Preventive medicine is organized through network of Institutes of Health, throughout the country. These institutes are also state-owned institutions, and are financed through contracts with the state health insurance fund.

The main streams of ongoing health reform in Serbia are:

● the introduction of licensing of physicians and accreditation of health facilities,

● the introduction of quality control system in health facilities

● and the rationalization of resources utilisation.

Although new laws on Health care and Chambers of health workers were passed in the parliament in December 2005, not all of these reform tracks are active up to now. The Chamber is in process of founding, and the Agency for accreditation is not yet founded. However, all health institutions have already formed Committees for quality management, and a system of quality indicators on a national level was introduced. In December 2005 the first benchmarking of hospitals in Serbia was made, based on the quality indicators.

One special reform track is particularly advanced: rationalization of drug utilization in hospitals. In 40 hospitals in Serbia (two-thirds of all hospitals) a medicines management system was introduced, with significant positive impact on both availability of drugs and utilization costs. This will also improve budgeting and financial management, as well as adding to the quality assurance targets for hospitals.

In the following text, a report on medicines management reform in Serbia is given, written by the two project coordinators, myself and Mr Tim Dodd, senior pharmacist, consultant of the Crown Agent project team, who implemented this project. The project was financed through grant assistance from the European Agency for Reconstruction, and the members of the project implementation team were: Professor Slobodan Jankovic, clinical pharmacologist, Mr Tim Dodd, senior pharmacist, Mr Jan Komrska, pharmacist and the Crown Agents Team leader, Dr Alexandar Spasic, Mr Dragan Bogavac, pharmacist, Mis. Natasa Moravcevic, pharmacist and Mrs. Branka Stojanovic, pharmacist.

Report on programme "Medicines Management in Hospitals in Serbia"
by Slobodan Jankovic and Tim Dodd

Introduction

"In all human activities, habits are acquired without much conscious thought and prescribing habits are no exception..Critical consideration of prescribing habits can help to improve them and need not be painful." Smith R. *BMJ* 1976

Medicines management is the term used to define the processes undertaken to ensure the selection, availability, and correct use of the medicines needed to treat effectively the patients of that hospital or institution. The classical method that has been promulgated in many areas is the formation of a Drug & Therapeutics Committee which determines a hospital formulary, or selected list of medicines, that can be made available for use by clinicians. This needs to be coupled with some form of audit or review of the use of medicines to ensure that the formulary is being complied with.

This classical method is seldom as successful as would be hoped, and there is some research to suggest that it actually increases costs elsewhere in the healthcare system, largely because it fails to engage clinicians in the process of selection and control of the use of medicines. There is a tension between those who make up the committee and those who actually treat the patients, resulting principally from the separation of the processes of selection and use of medicines. There is usually a significant delay between the prescribing of a medicine and the subsequent medicine use review, which severely reduces the value of the review. Finally, there can be an artificial authorization in the use of selected medicines arising specifically from there inclusion in the formulary. In addition therapeutic guidelines, while providing guidance and advice to clinicians, remain only guidelines and still require interpretation and implementation in respect of individual patient's needs.

The challenge, therefore, has been to combine the apparently conflicting issues of control of medicines and improving the choice and freedom of clinicians to prescribe appropriately for their patients; to increase the involvement of clinicians in the selection of treatment pathways; and to provide a useful and meaningful feedback to prescribers about their own use of medicines.

This programme, funded by EAR as part of a wider medicines management project and supported by the Ministry of Health, has introduced to selected hospitals across Serbia a system of medicines management that will achieve all of these objectives.

Medicines Management

There are four key components to the proposed medicine management system within hospitals:

1. Specialist Drug Lists or Unit Prescribing Policies

It may seem self evident that in order to be able to purchase and stock the medicines that will be required to treat patients, the hospitals need to know what will be required. Within each specialty therefore it is important to reach a consensus about how patients will be managed. It is unlikely that all eventualities can be foreseen, but the commonly treated diagnoses and conditions seen in each department are known and agreement can be reached by the specialists themselves about the best way to manage these. This choice of treatment modality will be informed by guidelines, research, experience, and shared objectives amongst the clinicians. At first this may simply be a list of the drugs most commonly used in that department (specialist drug list), but in time can be developed to form protocols, or treatment pathways (Unit Prescribing Policies).

2. Individual Patient Dispensing

Exactly as the name suggests this is a process by which medicines are dispensed each day specifically for individual patients and in sufficient quantity to meet the needs for that day. Additional arrangements are made for drug supply out with opening hours of the pharmacy department, but these are quite simple to organize and not onerous.

The process of supply is efficient in that it reduces wastage and reduces the amount of medicine resource that is in use at any time, since daily quantities instead of whole packs are dispensed. The dispensed medicines need to be labeled to identify the medicine and the patient to receive them and during this process of dispensing these medicines data are collected – patient, drug, dose, quantity, cost, date, diagnosis, doctor. These data are the keystone to this system. They can used to manage the stock of medicines, but also, and more importantly they are used to provide the reports on prescribing that are needed to review medicine usage.

3. Drug Charts

The prescribing of medicines currently taking place on the 'temperature lists' is fraught with problems. Temperature lists were designed to record temperature, blood pressure, and other physiological measures, and the addition of drug prescribing appears to be driven by an available piece of paper rather than any careful design.

The mixing of prescribing and the recording of physiological measures is not appropriate: many prescriptions are illegible, there is significant transcribing (with attendant errors) taking place, and there is a lack of continuity across different parts of the hospital where the patient is treated. Similarly, there is little standardization about the recording of the administration of the medicine to the patient, and in some places this is not done at all.

The introduction of the drug chart is intended to address all these issues and make the prescribing of medicines safer by reducing transcribing, while at the same time ensuring a record of the use of medicines in each patient. In this way there is a confidence that the patient is in fact receiving what the prescriber intended.

4. Drug & Therapeutic Committees

In this programme the role of this committee changes from being the committee that determines the drugs to be used, to that of a committee that ensures that medicines management takes place.

The processes for this will be described later, but in addition it is expected that the D&TC will determine the policies that are common across the hospital, for example antibiotics policy, disinfectant policy, hand washing policy, etc.

While it is easy to describe these components, it is their interaction and day to day practice that is important and will, in the final analysis deliver medicines management. The information collected about medicines use at the time of dispensing needs to be fed back to the specialists themselves and compared with the specialist drug lists they had previously identified as their needs. Did they treat the patents as they had intended? Is there significant deviation either as a whole or between clinicians? Was the initial drug list wrong or was the prescribing at fault? Most importantly, how are they going to correct any deviations? This review of their own prescribing needs to be reported to the hospital management, via the D&TC. In this way there is a 'freedom' by clinicians to prescribe appropriately for each patient, but there is also a responsibility to account to their peers for these choices.

The drug chart provides a place where therapy is prescribed and is written once and once only. No transcribing takes place and this chart goes with the patient wherever they are treated in the hospital so that each clinician can see the total therapy of the patient at the time they make a prescribing decision. This improves the security of that decision. In addition the record of the administration of the drug to the patient means that we can be certain that the patient received the intended therapy, which in turn helps to improve the management of the patient.

Dispensing individually for each patient not only improves efficiency, but also helps to ensure that the right drug is given to the right patient. This also provides the pharmacist the information needed to support more closely the clinicians in the management of the patients. At the time of dispensing the medicines the pharmacist has the information and opportunity to remind clinicians of their previously agreed treatment intentions, as well as being able to identify potential interactions or dosage problems, etc.

Far from being diminished the role of the D&TC is enhanced by being able to ensure the control of medicine use across the whole hospital without the necessity of lengthy and inefficient surveys. In this way control of medicines is improved without compromising the care of patients.

Progress in Hospitals in Serbia

An initial range of 40 hospitals across Serbia was identified in close cooperation of the Ministry of Health. Subsequently there has been some amendment to this as will be described later, but it is encouraging to be able to report that some hospitals not initially included have been actively seeking to adopt the procedures of medicines management.

In each case our approach has been to seek an initial meeting with the hospital director at which the principles, main components, and processes of medicines management have been described, as well as emphasizing that each hospital will need to identify and solve their own problems using the 'tools' and support that we can provide. In most cases this approach has been enthusiastically welcomed and often we have met with the whole management team.

Early in this process we recognized the important role the pharmacist will play in making the system work in each hospital. They are the only person who sees each prescription each day and the information needed for continuous review of prescribing arises directly from the pharmacy activities. Hospitals must have pharmacists with a supporting staff of technicians, etc., appropriately trained to meet these new challenges. With this in mind we commissioned the Faculty of Pharmacy, University of Belgrade to develop a post-graduate training course in Pharmaceutical Care. This is a distance-learning course, so pharmacists will not be absent from their work during the training, and will improve the pharmacists' contribution to the rational use of medicines in the hospitals. One critical factor in the further development of medicines management is the shortage of pharmacists working in hospitals.

In many hospitals we have made presentations/lectures about the principles, objectives, and strategy for medicines management. The purpose of these presentations is to introduce the concepts to the clinical staff of the hospital and to seek their support in making this process work in their hospital. We also take the opportunity to address some specific issue in prescribing, for example the appropriate use of antibiotics which is a major problem throughout Serbia.

All training sessions for the first presentations comprised of a lecture by Tim Dodd on the principles, objectives, and strategy for medicines management; a second lecture by Slobodan Jankovic outlining the results and experiences of using medicines management in hospitals; and finally a question and answer session. The second round of presentations utilized the same format, but focused on rational prescribing and antibiotic policies.

All presentations have been well received by participants and commented on by managers as bringing optimism, enthusiasm, and method to the problem of drug usage. In many hospital the presentations as well as forming part of the 'in-service' training of the hospitals, served to provide the necessary motivation and momentum to get people working on the medicines management issues within the hospitals.

Results

Each hospital has developed a D&TC which is the focus for medicines management activities within the hospital. These committees have encouraged clinicians to develop the specialist drug lists, identifying their specific requirements for the patients in each department or specialty. Antibiotics policies, including the use of antibiotics as prophylaxis in surgery and the restriction of critical antibiotics to cases of real need, have been developed in many of the hospitals and the remainder are being encouraged in this endeavour.

In each of the hospitals included in the project there has been identified at least one clinical area where IPD will be introduced. Where it is necessary, hospitals have created one or more satellite pharmacies so that IPD can take place closer to the patients. This improves the communication between clinicians and pharmacists and thus improves the service to patients. Computers and software, commissioned specifically for the purpose of IPD, have been supplied to each hospital through Crown Agents.

For those departments that will not yet benefit from IPD we are suggesting that a system of top-up of stock is introduced. This involves agreeing the range and quantity of stock to be held in the department. Twice or three times a week, more often for very busy departments, personnel from pharmacy come to the department to check the stock and top up to the agreed level. This system has the advantage improved management of the pharmacy workload, the pharmacist knows about all the stock in the hospital, it reduces total stock holding, and allows flexibility in sudden changes in drug usage.

The progress in each hospital differs partly due to the energy and enthusiasm focused on the project, but mainly due to the time they have been involved in the project. The Clinical Hospital Center in Kragujevac, where from the pilot project on medicine management originated, has established all elements of the system, achieving 100% coverage of total drug costs with the available drug budget transferred from Heath Insurance Fund; further development of the system is undertaken within the scope of current project, together with continuous monitoring of quality of the health services.

Early joiners, such as Cacak, Valjevo, Petrovac na Mlavi, Vranje, have already made significant improvement to their medicine usage and, with it, a reduction in the length of stay of the patient. The clear result is that there has been an improvement in the control of medicines without compromising the care of the patient.

It should be remembered, however, that 'savings' identified in these project hospitals may not result in financial savings. Rather they will allow purchase of medicines previously funded directly by the patients, or the purchase of a preferred choice of medicine previously unaffordable. The overall benefit is that the true cost of treatment of patients will be known and from this the funding required by hospitals can be calculated. Each hospital is encouraged to report progress quarterly using a specific form, in which they identify their own objectives and progress towards them.

One of the results of medicine management programme was a decrease in volume of drug utilization. This could be seen most clearly in the hospitals which joined the programme early.

Antibiotics account for the biggest share of drug budget in majority of Serbian hospitals. For example, hospital "Stefan Visoki" in Smederevska Palanka spent almost half of its budget in 2004 for antibiotics. Therefore, some of the hospitals, like Cacak, have put major effort to manage antibiotic use. The volume of antibiotic utilization decreased, primarily due to full implementation of preoperative antibiotic prophylaxis. A benefit that is not immediately apparent from this improved control of antibiotics is decrease in bacterial resistance to antibiotics, which will have a significant effect on public health of Serbia. The control is not based on cost but is focused on the effective use of antibiotics to ensure efficacy and avoid the development of resistant organisms, which are an increasing issue throughout the world.

Constraints

1) Changes in Management

This has been, and still is, a far reaching project and it requires, at the start, a lot of cooperation between the project team and the hospital management and staff. During the course of the project there has been a change in management in 12 of the hospitals we are working with. Each time this happens it is necessary to re-establish relationships and re-explain the project and its objectives. This lack of continuity is debilitating to the project and must have similar effect on all aspects of management and development in the hospitals.

2) Budgetary Management

A key requirement for all hospitals is that they can operate within their budgetary limits. However, in Serbia there appears to be little incentive for clinicians, themselves, to try to work within budgetary constraints. Indeed, there may be disincentives if the next year's budget is reduced in line with 'savings' made through more efficient use of medicines.

Figure 1. Comparison of total drug costs and antibiotic costs (in CSD) for year 2004 in hospital "Stefan Visoki" in Smederevska Palanka. The graph was made by the hospital's Chief pharmacist.

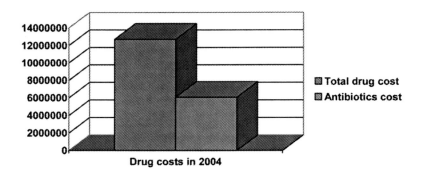

Table 1. Utilization of ceftriaxone (in DDD/1000 patient days) in three wards of Cacak hospital (Surgery + Orthopedics + Urology) during 5 different time periods. Antibiotic management started after period I. The table was supplied by the hospital programme implementation team.

Time period	I	II	III	IV	V
Ceftriaxone utilization (DDD/1000)	16.4	13.8	14.4	15.7	11.8

The data gained from the medicines management project should be used to estimate the true cost of treating patients and budgets agreed for expected patient loads and case-mix of each hospital. The only hospital which achieved operation within its budgetary limits in years 2003 and 2004 was the Clinical Hospital Centre in Kragujevac, but due only to persistent negotiations with Health Insurance Fund, based on precise data on actual workload and drug costs.

3) Pharmacy Staffing

It has been clear from the outset that there is a significant shortfall in the staff requirements for the pharmaceutical services in hospitals. This project has shown that the pharmacists are more than capable of ensuring the management of medicines within hospitals, but it is self-evident that they need to be there in sufficient numbers. A major initiative is required to attract more pharmacists into the hospital service, even if this means revising the salary structure or incentive schemes to make outlying hospital more attractive.

4) Clinical Pharmacologists

There is also a shortfall in the availability of advice and guidance from clinical pharmacologists in the development and assessment of clinical protocols. Constant review of prescribing and the identification of areas in need of guidelines and protocols is a major feature of medicines management and requires input from clinical pharmacologists. One solution would be for the clinical pharmacologists from the major centers and other hospitals fortunate to have this service, to be given formal links with those hospitals that do not have the service.

Conclusion

The overall conclusion is that the concepts of medicine management and the mechanisms required to achieve this have been readily and enthusiastically adopted within the hospitals of Serbia included in the project. The initial results suggest that this is a process that can be accepted by clinicians and will be sustainable in the future. The improved control of medicines not only improves the effectiveness of treatment, seen in the reduced length of stay, but increases public health through better use of antibiotics.

The shortage of pharmacists in hospitals needs to be addressed urgently to encourage more pharmacists to join the hospital service and ensure the continued successful management of medicines through the expansion of IPD and review of prescribing.

The Ministry of Health should encourage hospital managers in

Serbia to establish Clinical pharmacology departments in their hospitals, and use them as coordinating points for drug management process. The dissemination of improved medicine management to other hospitals in Serbia should be encouraged but needs to be matched by appropriate funding. The processes associated with medicines management and the reporting of progress could easily be incorporated into the quality assurance reports of the hospitals and healthcare institutions, thus giving the Ministry an assurance that the use of medicines is under control.

REFERENCES/BIBLIOGRAPHY

1 The law on health insurance. *Official Gazette of Republic of Serbia* 2005; 107: 48 – 92.
2 The law on chambers of health workers. *Official Gazette of Republic of Serbia* 2005; 107: 96 – 104.
3 The law on health care. *Official Gazette of Republic of Serbia* 2005; 107: 112 – 161.
Vrca VB, Bo□ikov V, Crncec MN, Sutli? □, Šimic D, Becirevic M.Uticaj primene sustava raspodele jedinicne terapije na potrošnju lijekova.Lijec Vjesn 2000; 122:110-8.
U.S. General Accounting Office: *Unit Dose Life Cycle Costs Analysis and Application to a Recently Constructed Health Care Facility. Study of Health Facilities Construction Costs.* A Report to the Congress by the United States General Accounting Office,1972.
Brown TR. *Handbook of Institutional Pharmacy Practice*, 3rd., Williams & Wilkins, Baltimore,1991;165-73.
Slater WE, Jacobsen R, Hripko JR et al. Unit dose drops expenses. *Hospital* 1972; 46:88-94.
Bergman U, Christenson I, Jansson B, Winholm BE. Auditing hospital drug utilization by means of defined daily doses per bed-day. A methodological study. *Eur J Clin Pharmacol* 1980;17;183-7.
WHO Collaborating Centre for Drug Statistics Methodology. ATC Index with DDD's 1998. Oslo,1998.
Minor MF. Justifying the cost of unit dose system without reliance on saving of nursing. *Hosp Pharm* 1975;10:97-9.
Hendrix FL. The administrator of a small hospital looks at unit dose system. *Hosp Form Mgt* 1973;9:11-3.
Black HJ,Tester WW. Decentralised pharmacy operations utilising the unit dose concept. *Am J Hosp Pharm* 1963;21:334-50.
Laing RO, Hogerzeil HV, Ross-Degnan D. Ten recommendations to improve use of medicines in developing countries. *Health Policy and Planning* 2001; 16(1): 13–20.
WHO. *How to develop and implement a national drug policy.* 2nd edition. Geneva: World Health Organization, 2001.
WHO. *Guide to Good Prescribing. A practical manual.* Geneva: World Health Organization, 1994.
Jankovic SM, Dukic Dejanovic S. Drug utilization trends in clinical hospital center

"Kragujevac" from 1997 to 1999. *Indian J Pharmacol* 2001; 33: 29-36.

Jankovic SM, Vasic LjM, Maksimovic MR, Cupurdija VB, Kostic IR, Kovacevic ZN. An analysis of drug use indicators in primary care health facilities operating in the city of Kragujevac. *General Practice* 1999; 1-14. (http://www.priory.com/fam/Kosovo.htm)

Flores W, Ochoa H, Briggs J, Garcia R, Kroeger A. Economic costs associated with inadequate drug prescribing: an exploratory study in Chiapas, Mexico. *Acta Trop* 2003; 88(1): 57-68.

Lee EK, Malone DC. Comparison of peptic-ulcer drug use and expenditures before and after the implementation of a government policy to separate prescribing and dispensing practices in South Korea. *Clin Ther* 2003; 25(2): 578-92.

Das B, Sarkar C, Datta A, Bohra S. A study of drug use during pregnancy in a teaching hospital in western Nepal. *Pharmacoepidemiol Drug Saf* 2003; 12(3): 221-5.

Adigun AQ, Ishola DA, Akintomide AO, Ajayi AA. Shifting trends in the pharmacologic treatment of hypertension in a Nigerian tertiary hospital: a real-world evaluation of the efficacy, safety, rationality and pharmaco-economics of old and newer antihypertensive drugs.

Sweden: universal welfare versus market mechanisms and privatization

Gunnar Ågren and Susanne Öhrling

The objectives of the health care sector are of decisive importance: is the objective to accomplish health or to offer services to groups of care-consumers? The only reasonable assumptions for medical interventions is that the system aims to deliver improved health and quality of life.

Current knowledge suggests that a health care system that is primary care based, and easily accessible for all without economic restrictions, is the best form of organization to deliver these objectives.

A historical background

Access to free, basic medical care is an ancient demand from the working-class movement.

A landmark in the establishment of this style of system came after World War II – when the British Labour government in 1948, implementing the principles of the Beveridge Report, established the National Health Service (NHS) which was free at point of use for all health care, including dental care and glasses.

In Sweden, the equivalent to the Beveridge Reports was the 1943 Inquiry of Axel Höjer (head of the Medical Board 1935-52), which proposed universal free health care in Sweden: but as in Britain, the doctors' association, the Swedish Medical Association, opposed it. They partly wanted to keep the possibility of charging the patients and partly to keep the focus on hospital-based care. Eventually, as in Britain, the doctors made a compromise with the government, which involves the continuation of a large private sector in outpatient care, as well as private beds in hospitals.

Primary care and mental health services are a state responsibility, with regional councils taking responsibility for hospital care. Universal health insurance was introduced in 1955, but a low, universal fee for use of all health services – the '7-crown reform' – was introduced in 1971.

There was a strong development of the health care system until 1990, although with more emphasis on hospital care than primary care. But a neo-liberal ideological offensive in the 1980s brought steps towards the introduction of a health care market, with the 'purchaser/ provider split' being introduced in many regions.

Until this point in time a publicly-financed and provided health care, distributed according to need, was considered good. But the neoliberals introduced the idea that productivity was too low in the public sector, and that the market would create a more flexible and effective health care. The same assumptions inspired theories of new public management (lean production) – despite the fact that all experience suggested the opposite– the market created a less effective and less efficient health care system.

Eventually a number of County Councils were persuaded to try to create artificial markets by making a division between 'purchaser' and 'provider' of care, and by putting price-tags on different kinds of treatments: some parts of the health care sector were contracted out to private companies.

International development

In 1978 the WHO enacted the declaration of Alma Ata, which set the goal of Health For All, embraced the values of universalism, and pleaded for a population based primary care. A number of developing countries tried to construct locally rooted health care systems, often using professionals other than doctors.

This was counteracted by the USA and strong professional interests wanting to reduce the efforts to a few basic interventions, such as vaccinations and giving saline to infants with diarrhea.

The Structural Adjustment Policy (SAP) operated by the World Bank and IMF contributed to the demolition of these primary care based systems – and became a contributing cause of the AIDS-catastrophe in many poor countries.

There were also economic constraints on health services, and cost control became a major problem, with severe cut-backs and a worsening of the work environment for health workers The market system also meant that groups with lesser resources experienced even more difficulties in getting access to care – and this was an important factor for the crisis within psychiatry.

During the second half of the 1990s, the market-style system of health care developed a bad reputation: the purchaser/provider model was abandoned by several county councils. However the international offensive continued, with big international companies seeking to join the Swedish health care market, triggering a debate over for-profit hospitals.

The current situation

The beginning of the current decade has seen new initiatives to promote privatization, with the main arguments centred on:

■ Alleged low standards in public sector care.

■ Lack of influence of service users.

■ The need for 'freedom of choice'.

Eventually there was a counter offensive from the left, which brought a return in some regions to an ordinary budget system. A new government bill, supported by the Social Democrats, Left party, and the Green party, was opposed by all the right wing parties, because it:

■ Prohibits new for-profit hospitals, and

■ Prevents publicly funded hospitals taking patients paid by private insurance.

The main arguments against a market in health care are well-established:

■ Cost control is more difficult.

■ Contracts with private providers make it more difficult to adapt health services to changing needs, and for patients and commissioners to choose between providers.

■ Preventive activities receive much lower priority and resourcing.

■ The total burden of adjustment falls on the remaining public sector in health care.

■ The competence of the organisations purchasing care is not enough to control different providers of care.

■ There is a risk that private finance could be introduced.

■ Other groups with interests in health care may became provider (i.e. the drug industry)

From a public health perspective, the main problems arising from a market-style system are slightly different:

■ Reduced accessibility due to high fees

■ Increasing costs of drugs

■ Difficulty in controlling total costs in a market system with a large number of providers

■ Problems introducing preventive policies

■ Lack of cooperation with other sectors in society, especially in rehabilitation

Elements essential for a health promoting health system include a good primary care system with a responsibility for the whole population, accessible at a reasonable cost and with the capacity to work with prevention. Any shortcomings in primary care have to be paid for in other parts of the health services, or in society as a whole

However market-like conditions have made it difficult enforce preventive activities, and it has also been very hard to put a market price on preventive activities – especially primary prevention and activities directed to underprivileged groups.

The economic crisis during the 1990s further increased these problems.

An additional problem has been the medicalisation of prevention, with a tendency to use drugs to compensate for an unhealthy life-style: for instance antihypertensive drugs, antidepressants and lipid-lowering drugs may be used in some cases instead of other preventive activities.

Moreover the very strong marketing of drugs may lead to lack of cost-effectiveness in the total health system. It is hard to protect health care against other interests, as pharmaceutical companies gain increased power and thus gain additional possibilities for to control health care and health policy.

There are other contradictory forces which also tend to undermine public health and health policies at national and international level.

On an international scale there can be conflicts between trade policy, agricultural policy and health policy – especially regarding recommendations on consumption of alcohol, tobacco and food.

Health policy can also conflict with strong economic interests, and with the need for state revenues – for example in the extent to which governments seek to limit and control harmful gambling.

Other factors, such as rising unemployment, economic insecurity and inequity may create problems which are impossible to counteract from the health sector, even though these problems clearly influence the health sector. Health policy must therefore be a part of general economic and social policy.

There are a number of these problems also in Sweden today, bringing an immense strain on the health care system in the future.

Health services have to be distributed according to need, not on the basis of the demands of economically and socially influential groups. They have to be based on a strong and accessible primary care.

While the public sector is often regarded as bureaucratic and lacking in influence in achieving public health goals, a large private sector, and strong market mechanisms in health care are in conflict with planning, prioritisation and prevention on the basis of needs.

It is not sufficient to discuss the organisation of the health care system, it is also important to discuss the content of the poilicy, and to have a strategy and goals, with the target always being centred on better health for the population.

Health policy in Turkey in the context of the "Right to Health" and "Privatisation"

Fatih Artvinli

For the last 20 years, Turkish society has been faced with a schedule for completely commercialising the health sector. Since 1978 Turkey has been subjected to numerous stand-by agreements of the International Monetary Fund (IMF). In each case, Turkey was required to transform itself to conform to neo-liberal prerequisites.

Starting from the early 1980s, Turkish governments began to give generous subsidies to the private health care market. These subsidies took different forms such as their exemption from customs taxes, cash grants and supporting grants. One other form of subsidy given to the private health care market was in the form of increased expenditure by the public health care sector in the private health care market.

The Ministry of Health Hospitals increased their spending on medical supplies from the private medical industry. Public sector health providers such as State Hospitals, University Hospitals and Social Insurance Institution hospitals also transferred ancillary services, such as cleaning, security and laboratory services, to the private market.

The years between 1980 and 2000 were the 'period of active privatisation', during which the governments adopted a more 'neo-liberal' perspective which viewed healthcare and social security as services whose price would be determined in the marketplace on the basis of the principles of supply and demand.

The victory of the Justice and Development Party (JDP) in the 2001 elections signified the beginning of a new era. The JDP moderated and realigned its political discourse on the basis of a neo-liberal model, with a populist and conservative tone.

The government agreed to continue the adjustment program signed with the IMF, along the lines of its predecessors. Since then, the government has been actively pursuing an agenda of economic liberalisation and privatisation of state economic enterprises. It is in this context that health sector reform has re-emerged on the political agenda.

The JDP government announced its reform program, 'Transformation in Health', in December 2003. The 'Transformation of Health' program declared that its central objective in the reform was "establishing a qualified and effective health system to which everybody can have access."

But in practice we saw the real face of the reform:

The essence of the changes in health sector the conversion of public health institutions into commercial enterprises, directing public health expenditures towards the private sector and gradually privatising all health services.

In this period, total health expenditures have been increased from US $11 billion to US $19 billion. However most of these expenditures were in the form of medicine and service purchased from the private sector. While 24% of health expenditures were from private sector in the year 2000, this percentage exceeded 50% in 2005.

On the other hand, the percentage of preventive health services within total health expenditures has been reduced from 5% to 2.6% for the last 5 years. For example, between 2002 and 2004, the percentage covered by measles vaccination has fallen. The percentage of BCG vaccination is still less than it was in 2001.

Another destructive effect of commercialisation is in the program on tuberculosis control. The chance of tuberculosis patients deriving benefit from commercialized public health institutions is reduced, and the tuberculosis control program, which has already had very significant problems, has entered a more threatening phase.

Now let us look at the structural changes in health policy in three steps:

The first step was the transfer of the ownership of Social Insurance Institution (SII) hospitals to the Ministry of Health. This was a step towards setting up a health insurance system which gathers all health insurance tasks under a single umbrella. These tasks previously belonged to different social security institutions. The SII was an institution which delivered low-cost services to a large mass of people, giving medicines to workers. This role of the SII was the most serious obstacle to the commercialisation of health services in both practical and legal terms. The transfer of SII hospitals to Ministry of Health has indirectly paved the way for a rapid privatization of health sector.

Then civil servants were given the 'opportunity' to benefit from private health services. In this process, the government began to exploit the long-established image of 'good private hospitals versus bad public hospitals'. In this context, there has been a serious transfer of resources to the private sector. The crucial point in this process is that because the contribution of the state to their health expenditure was limited, civil servants have had to pay higher fees, exceeding their personal budgets, to obtain 'higher quality' medical services.

During the process of joint usage of hospitals attached to the Ministry of Health and Social Insurance Institution, the government has used a populist discourse such as:

"the end of queues in SII hospitals"; "SII members now getting their chance to apply to private health institutions like civil servants"(!); and "the opportunity for SII members to buy their medicines from any pharmacy shop."

Health expenditures have increased, but as you might guess, the pharmaceutical firms have been the most satisfied ones, because spending on drugs has increased by 47 %.

The second step of reform was the introduction of a performance-based remuneration system in all institutions attached to the Ministry of Health, through a directive on extra payments from revolving funds. Under this directive, physicians are to be given marks for services they deliver and the performance of each physician is to be evaluated on the basis of these marks.

This practice, which completely disregards the specific nature of health care services, further weakens solidarity among health workers and gives rise to a situation which is ethically questionable. This performance-based remuneration system aims for the internalization of a private sector mentality in public health.

What lies at the basis of this mentality is the maximization of profit, so the relationship between the doctor and the patient is transferred to a relationship between the doctor and his client.

The third step involves the family health care system which was imposed by IMF and World Bank. A law has already been passed to launch a pilot scale implementation of this system. Again we see the populism of the government.

In Duzce, as a pilot region for family health care system, the government began to give health services free of charge, funded from the money given by World Bank. But in a larger context, the family health care system lays the ground for a competitive environment where physicians will deliver their services while upholding their concerns for keeping clients. The system as a whole tends to over-utilise medicine and medical technology. A lot of European countries have given up using this model and other countries are still debating over it.

Taken together, these arrangements define each provider delivering health care services (whether at primary or secondary level) as a competitive agent, bound to compete in a market-oriented environment.

Thus, some of the most important properties of public service, such as being nonprofit oriented, financing the service from budget, and giving service through public officials, are abrogated. With these arrangements, it is very obvious that the 'social' characteristics of the health service will be removed drastically, and health care will be transformed into a commodity.

Another development in health policy is the Social Security Reform, which was approved by the parliament two weeks ago. The basic aim of the reform is to reduce the state's contributions to social security. Some of the key elements include a reduction in pension income, an increase in the age of retirement and an increase in payments for health services.

The Social Security Reform has also brought many changes which work to the disadvantage of employees and needy people. Instead of providing social security funding from a national budget which is composed of taxes taken according to individuals' income, the reform agrees to provide social security services according to the basis of premium payments. The payment level of premium for employees to retire, will gradually be increased from 7000 days to 9000 days. More than 60% of working men in Turkey are unregistered employees, and Turkey is one of the countries where inequality of income distribution is among the highest in the world. Unfortunately, our country is getting ready to sacrifice social security in the name of social security reform.

In any case, provisions in the new laws warn citizens that they may be ineligible for insurance, if they fail to pay attention to their personal health! However citizens are of course free to subscribe from their personal incomes to supplementary insurance agencies that will offer cover above this minimum guaranteed package.

According to the general health insurance law, everybody must pay the premiums, even retired people. If you miss out on paying the premiums for three months you can not get health services.

So health will not be a right – instead it will be a service that you can buy if you have money.

When one considers that one-fifth of population in Turkey has no health insurance cover, the threat becomes clear.

As we have shown, we face a process of step by step privatisation of public health services in Turkey. These measures are not unique to Turkey or health sector. We need to know that this is a broad and complex problem of neo-liberalism in general.

The neo-liberal approach transforms basic concepts, defining access to health care as an issue of personal responsibility, not a public responsibility. We need a complete change of paradigm to restore the right to health as a universal human right.

The results of health reform in Turkey: increased and deepened inequalities

Onur Hamzaoglu and Feride Sacaklioglu

used to have and le best infant and maternal mortality rate

ABSTRACT

There used to be a well defined, population based, public primary health care system in Turkey. Health was a social right which was gained at birth and health services were the responsibility of the state.

The last crisis of the capitalist system had an impact on the social and economic policies of Turkey through the January 24th decisions and the September 12th 1980 military coup d'état. Economic and social life has been reorganised according to the structural adjustment programs of the IMF and the interests of the national and international forces of capital.

As the result of this reorganisation, debt increased and the balance of income distribution has changed – in favour of the upper classes. Taxes on the upper classes decreased while indirect taxes became the main resource of the budget. The share of rent, interest and profit in the national income increased, whereas the share of salaries decreased. The public sector, including health services and education, has continued to be privatised since the mid 1980s in Turkey.

Public funds for health care have decreased within this framework. The effect was the hidden privatisation of the hospital care. Hospitals are pushed to survive on their revolving funds. Public guaranteed health care started to transform itself to private health care, even in public institutions. Health is accepted as a commodity for sale in the market.

Two World Bank funded health projects were the driving force of privatisation during the 1990s. Although the governments have changed, there has been no change in the attack on public health care. The most recent step has been the privatisation of primary health care since 2000.

During the last 25 years, due to the changes of economic and social policies, the inequities in health (infant and child mortality, antenatal care, hospital based deliveries, immunisation, contraceptive use, distribution of doctors, midwives and health centers) between urban and rural areas, between regions and classes have increased. One of the results is the lack of health care services in over ten thousand villages.

Unless the economic policies, economic inequities and privatisation of health care are changed, the inequities in health will increase.

BACKGROUND

This article concentrates on the concept of health. The background factors and the history of so called "health reform" are discussed in order to define what should be done for a healthy society.

There is a regression in terms of social rights in all central and peripheral capitalist countries. The reason for this regression is the current crisis of capitalism which began at the end of the 1960s, and the economic policies introduced in order to combat it.

All the social issues have been excluded from the social distribution area. During this process the uprising of the working class is inhibited through ideological means.

This process which began with the 1980s military coup d'etat in Turkey is based on the rules and necessities of the central capitalist countries, and the national bourgeoisie acts as the subcontractor of the international capital. The health sector, like other areas of social policy has tried to adopt the rules of the market. The relatively profitable areas of the social sector are opened up as an investment area for national and international capital.

The health policies and the targets of the health sectors that have been defined by several governments since the 1980s are not different from each other. The same models of financial and service organisation are offered to the peripheral capitalist countries by the World Bank, the International Monetary Fund and the WHO.

The working class has still an opportunity to invert this process, although they seem ideologically defeated.

INTRODUCTION

Health is not an individual matter: it is the result of social conditions. For that reason, health should be evaluated in a social context, with its all determinants – including economic, political and cultural.

Health is being able to produce in order to respond to necessities equally, and to protect the biological and mental wholeness and to improve this wholeness through social organisation and collective production processes[1]. For that reason health should be considered as an output of the relationships of producers and production.

The concept of health covers all of the areas of a human being's labour and life. Health services are not sufficient for being healthy. Simultaneously, nutrition, shelter, education, transportation, environment, work, recreational, social and cultural activities are directly related to the health of society.

The richness of a country is not a guarantee of the health of society, unless the wealth is distributed equally. The socialist countries had better levels of health than richer capitalist countries. Within the capitalist system the level of health is better in the countries where the social services, including the health services, are provided by public sector. The determining factor is the production and distribution relationships[2].

Treatment of patients is not the sole priority. Preventive services should be included within the organisation of health care.

1.1. Who is the owner of health reform? [4]

It is well known that attempts have been made since the 1980s to change the health care system. The direction of this change is towards the market: in other words a system based on the demands of the social classes that determine the distribution of resources in this new model. They are not only intervening in the health sector, but also in education, local government, public administration, universities, the working environment, social security, the national treasury, and forestry.

Furthermore, these interventions that we are witnessing are not limited to Turkey. This approach is the result of the "Washington Consensus" of the World Bank and International Monetary Fund, and their structural adjustment policies. Many countries have adapted these policies against their wishes.

There are three main objectives of these policies.

● First is the dominance of the rules of the market;

● second is limiting the services given by the public sector,

● and the third is limitation of the public regulative function.

The governments of the central capitalist countries in Europe provided social security, job security, unemployment insurance and a secure retirement to their citizens from 1945 until around 25 years ago.

Starting in the 1970s, because of the depression of capitalism, profit ratios started to decline and governments tried to get rid of their social responsibilities, to reduce the cost of the labour, and abandoned welfare state policies. At this period of time health expenditures were one third of total social expenditures.

Demographic changes, technological improvements and wider usage of technology, exponential increases in drug prices and raised expectations of health services combined to increase the cost of health care, and health expenditures increased more rapidly than the increase in national income[3].

The bourgeoisie abdicated the responsibility for reproducing the labour force which they had undertaken before the crisis, and themselves broke the social peace.

The structural adaptation policies were imposed by WB and IMF on behalf of the international capital, in order to maximise their profit. They use different tools to attack.

The first tool is wars. The USA has for decades created wars in the Middle East, Africa, Balkans, Afghanistan, and Iraq, in order to increase exploitation and reinforce the hegemony of the imperialist powers. It seems like they will continue creation of wars in Syria, Iran and wherever possible. Where capitalism has militarised its economy the capitalists maximise their profit through wars.

The second tool is the restructuring of the state, in which the state should abandon its responsibilities; all the public properties would be sold to the private sector for nothing. There will be a gradual privatisation both ownership and the fields of service of public responsibilities such as education, health services, etc.

The third mechanism is through dissolving the trade unions, flexible production approaches and lower wages, diminishing the cost of the labour force. They established the legal structure and background and through their ideological struggle they have deceived the workers into accepting diminished social rights.

1.2. What is the aim of Health Reforms? [4]

The aims of the reforms could be summarised as follows.

The responsibility of the state in the field of health will be diminished to a regulator rather than service provider for the working classes.

There is a dramatic decrease in the share of the general budget in health expenditures. Out of pocket payments, co-payments and insurance fees would finance the health care instead of general budget. That means it will become legal to provide health care to the people who have money and in accordance with their ability to pay.

Patients will become customers, and unprofitable items such as preventive care will be excluded from the service spectrum of the private health sector.

The health sector is fragmented between providers and purchasers, and the relationship between the two is determined by the dynamics of the market economy. Through creating competition they aim to purchase health services more cheaply. This approach is not rational: as UK experience shows us that this approach has made the service more expensive.

Even public health services will be commercialised and forced to work on the basis of a market. Public institutions will be forced to survive on their revolving funds. Their competitive power will be reduced day by day in the face of national and international capital, and many public hospitals will inevitably be closed. The health market will fall under the control of the big hospital chains; a monopoly of health care will be established. This will result in service packages which diminish the right to health through.

Health staff are forced to work on the basis of performance based and part time contracts. At the same time the rights of health staff are neglected.

1.3. Health Reform: which government's program? [5]

None of these policies is the invention of the current government. All the governments since 1980s are acting as the subcontractors of the attack waged by capital through WB and IMF programs. The main principles of these programs were the same, although their promises and voters seemed different. Their hidden aim was to overcome the long crisis of capitalism by reshaping the health sector in accordance the interest of the bourgeoisie.

As in many countries, WB loaned US$ 348 million to Turkey: most of this finance has been paid to the supervisors that WB recommended.

Through the years all of the government programs were more or less the same: the governments blame this similarity on the problems experienced in the health sector.

METHOD

Data from the Turkish National Health Survey has been used. Two measures have been used in order to demonstrate the inequalities in health. The first measure is the Rate Ratio and the second measure is the Population Attributable Risk. The Rate ratio is calculated by dividing the rates of lowest versus highest socioeconomic status-groups. Population Attributable Risk (%) is calculated as the difference between the overall rate and the rate for the highest socioeconomic group, expressed as a percentage of the overall rate.

The population-attributable risk not only reflects the morbidity and mortality rates of lower socioeconomic groups as compared with the highest socioeconomic group but also their population size: the larger the groups with high rates, the larger the potential reduction in overall rates is.

This measure can be interpreted as the proportional reduction in overall morbidity and mortality rates that would occur in the hypothetical case that everyone experiences the rates of the highest socioeconomic group.

FINDINGS

As shown in Table 1, the Infant Mortality Rate was 134 per thousand live births in 1978, where in the year 2003 this data fell to 29 per thousand live births. But when rural and urban IMRs were compared; for one infant death in urban areas there were 1.2 and 1.7 infant deaths in the years 1978 and 2003 respectively. Similarly, there were 1.4 and 1.9 infant deaths in rural areas compared to one death in urban areas in the years 1978 and 2003 respectively. In other words, if the rural areas could reach the socio-economic level of urban areas in 1978, 11.2% of infant deaths could be prevented. However, preventable infant deaths were 20.7% by 2003. Comparing the west and east of the country; if the socio-economic level of the country could reach the level of the west, in 1978 19.4% and in 2003 27.6% of the infant deaths could be prevented.

When the mother's education is considered, more infants died whose mothers were less educated. There were 1.68 and 1.56 infant deaths of less educated mothers for one infant death of more educated mothers by the year 1993 and 1998 respectively. By the year 2003 this ratio is 2.83

when mothers educated for eight years or more were compared with uneducated mothers.

As demonstrated in figure 1, if the uneducated mothers' educational level could be improved to the level of at least primary education, then 17.1% and 37.9% of the infant deaths could be prevented respectively. If the socio-economic level of the country could reach to the level of the west, in 1978 19.4% and in 2003 27.6% of the infant deaths could be prevented.

Another criterion is the percentage of malnourished children aged under five. There were 18.9% and 12.2% stunted children in the years of 1993 and 2003 respectively. But there are inequalities between urban

Table 1: Infant Mortality Rate according to years, residence, demographic region and inequality indicators[6-12]

	1978	1983	1988	1993	1998	2003
Residence						
Urban	119.0	67.4	50.1	44.0	35.2	23.0
Rural	146.0	128.3	105.7	65.4	55.0	39.0
Rural/Urban(RR)	1.23	1.90	2.11	1.49	1.56	1.70
PAR(%)	11.2				17.6	20.7
Demographic Region						
West	108.0	82.5	44.5	42.7	32.8	22.0
South	109.0	-	96.3	55.4	32.7	29.0
Central	151.0	97.6	90.0	57.9	41.3	21.0
North	141.0	112.5	-	44.2	42.0	34.0
East	147.0	137.4	103.0	60.0	61.5	41.0
East/West(RR)	1.36	1.67	2.32	1.41	1.88	1.86
PAR(%)	19.4	18.8	42.7	18.8	23.4	27.6
Mother's Education						
No education/ Primary incomplete				68.0	60.5	No education/ Primary incomplete 51.0
Primary school and above				43.6	36.1	First level primary 25.0
						Second level primary and ↑18.0
↓ primary/↑primary (RR)				1.56	1.68	↓ primary / ↑ high school 2.83
PAR				17.1	15.5	37.9
Total	134.0	101.6	77.7	52.6	42.7	29.0

and rural, west and east and according to the years. There were 1.7 stunted children in rural areas for one stunted child in urban areas by 1993. This is increased by 2003 to 2.0 stunted children. When the regions considered, in 1993 for each stunted child in the west there were 3.3 stunted children in the east and this is unfortunately increased to 4.1 stunted children by 2003.

From another point of view; 21.7% and 26.2% of the malnutrition could be prevented in 1993 and 2003 respectively if socio-economic conditions of rural and urban areas were equal. Similarly 46.0% and 54.9% of the malnutrition could be prevented in 1993 and 2003 respectively if socio-economic conditions of west and east were equal. When the mother's education is considered, children under five years old whose mothers were less educated were more stunted. While the percentage of stunted children was decreasing in the country, the conditions of the children of less educated mothers worsened. There is an increase in inequalities.

According to the data in the figure 2; if the uneducated mothers' educational level could be improved to the level of at least primary education. 76.7% and 76.2% of the stunted children could be prevented in

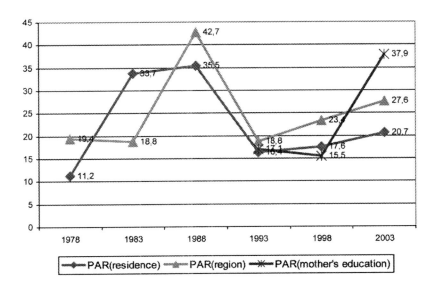

Figure 1: Infant Mortality Rate and PAR comparisons according to Residence, Demographic Region and Mother's Education[6-12]

Table 2: Stunted Children (-2SD↓) according to years, residence, demographic region and inequality indicators[9-12]

	1993	1998	2003
Residence	%		%
Urban	14.8	12.6	9.0
Rural	25.2	22.0	18.4
Rural/Urban(RR)	1.70	1.75	2.04
PAR(%)	21.7	21.3	26.2
Demographic Region	%		%
West	10.2	9.9	5.5
South	14.8	13.5	10.4
Central	18.8	11.6	9.5
North	12.9	12.8	13.0
East	33.3	30.0	22.5
East/West(RR)	3.27	3.03	4.09
PAR(%)	46.0	38.1	54.9
Mother's Education			
No education/ Primary incomplete	30.3	31.0	No education/ Primary incomplete 25.3
Primary school	14.9	11.8	First level primary 9.0
Above primary school	4.4	4.0	Second level primary 5.6
			High school and higher 2.9
↓ primary/↑primary (RR)	6.89	7.75	↓ primary / ↑ high school 8.72
PAR	76.7	75.0	76.2
Total	**18.9**	**16.0**	**12.2**

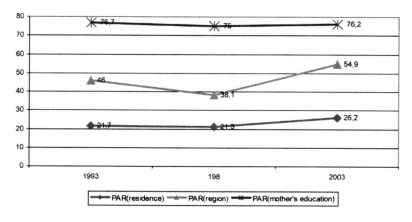

Figure 2: Stunted Children and PAR comparisons according to Residence, Demographic Region and Mother's Education[9-12]

1993 and 2003 respectively. If the socio-economic level of the rural areas could reach to the level of the urban areas, in 1978 22% and in 2003 26% of the stunted children could be prevented.

In 1983 58.0% and in 2003 22.7% of births occurred outside of health care institutions. For each delivery which occurred outside of health care institutions in urban areas, 2.1 and 2.5 births occurred in rural areas in the same conditions by 1983 and 2003 respectively. Again for each birth that occurred outside of health care institutions in the west there were 2.3 and 5.4 births in the east. From a more general point of view, if the socio-economic levels of rural and urban areas were equaled, 36.2% and 36.6% of the deliveries that occurred outside of health care institutions could be prevented. Similarly if the west and east of the country were equaled, 36.2% and 62.6% of the deliveries that occurred outside of health care institutions could be prevented (Table3).

Table 3: Deliveries occurred outside of health care according to residence, demographic region and inequality indicators[7-12]

	1983	1988	1993	1998	2003
Residence (%)					
Urban	37.0	27.6	27.5	19.8	14.4
Rural	76.0	52.8	59.5	40.3	35.7
Rural/Urban(RR)	2.05	1.91	2.16	2.04	2.48
PAR(%)	36.2	29.4	31.9	28.0	36.6
Demographic Region (%)					
West	37	27.6	19.8	13.4	8.5
South	67	45.2	37.2	30.8	21.5
Central	49	34.9	36.0	16.7	11.8
North	63	24.5	35.9	16.3	14.7
East	84	63.1	69.8	55.6	45.6
East/West(RR)	2.27	2.29	3.53	4.15	5.36
PAR(%)	36.2	37.3	51.0	51.3	62.6
Mother's Education (%)					
No education/ Primary incomplete			66.0	55.5	No education/ Primary incomplete 51.7
Primary school			29.3	19.6	First level primary 13.8
Above primary school			12.0	3.8	Second level primary 6.7
					High school and higher 3.2
↓ primary/↑primary (RR)			5.5	14.6	↓ primary / ↑ high school 16.2
PAR			70.3	86.2	85.9
Total	58.0	39.1	40.4	27.5	22.7

When pregnant women are considered, although there is a slight improvement over the years, there are differences according to the educational level. In the last ten years the less educated women could not benefit from this improvement, and the difference between educated and uneducated women increased. Uneducated mothers were six times more likely to have deliveries outside of health care institutions in 1983 – increasing to 15 times more likely in 1998 and to 16 in 2003 – than educated mothers.

As demonstrated in figure 3 if the uneducated mothers' level of education could be increased to the level of educated mothers, in 1993 70.3% of the deliveries, and in 2003 85.9% of the deliveries that occurred outside of health care institutions could be prevented. If all the demographic regions of the country could be equaled with the west of the country, in 1983 36% and in 2003 63% of them could be prevented.

Another health service evaluation criterion is the level of fully immunised 12-23 months old children. In 1998 54.3% and in 2003 45.8% of children were not fully immunised (Table 4). In the same years there were 1.3 and 1.7 children not fully immunised in eastern Turkey for each

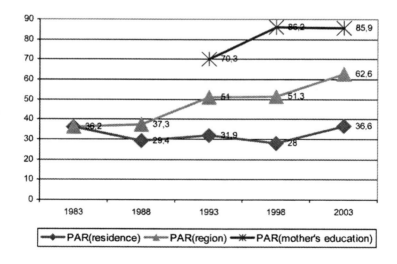

Figure 3: Deliveries Occurred Outside of Health Care and PAR comparisons according to Residence, Demographic Region and Mother's Education[7-12]

Table 4: Un-immunized 12-23 months old children according to residence, demographic region and inequality indicators[9-12]

	1993	1998	2003
Residence (%)			
Urban	25.7	48.2	37.1
Rural	49.1	63.2	63.5
Rural/Urban(RR)	1.91	1.31	1.71
PAR(%)	27.2	11.2	19.0
Demographic Region (%)			
West	24.0	49.8	27.0
South	18.9	42.7	39.8
Central	34.1	48.2	39.0
North	36.8	41.1	39.9
East	59.4	77.1	65.2
East/West(RR)	2.48	1.55	2.41
PAR(%)	46.5	24.3	41.0
Mother's Education (%)			
No education/ Primary incomplete	52.0	71.5	No education/ Primary incomplete 73.9
Primary school	29.1	52.0	First level primary 39.1
Above primary school	16.4	36.0	Second level primary 38.8
			High school and higher 31.5
↓ primary/↑primary (RR)	3.17	1.99	↓ primary / ↑ high school 2.35
PAR	53.5	33.7	31.2
Total	**35.3**	**54.3**	**45.8**

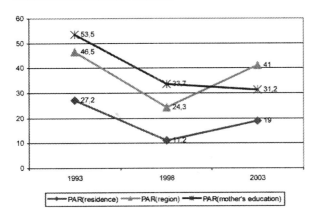

Figure 4: Un-immunized 12-23 months old children and PAR comparisons according to Residence, Demographic Region and Mother's Education[9-12]

child in western Turkey. If the rural areas were equaled to urban areas 11.2% and 19.0% of the children could be fully immunised respectively. Similarly, if the whole country could have the same socio-economic conditions of the western Turkey, 24.3% of children in 1998 and 41.0% in 2003 could be fully immunised (Table 4).

The ratio among the uneducated and educated mothers' children was one to three by 1993. This ratio decreased in favor of uneducated mothers' children to 1.99 by 1998, but increased to 2.35 by 2003. In general although the ratio of un-immunised children decreased through the time, uneducated mothers' children are still disadvantaged.

As demonstrated in figure 4; in 2003 if the mothers' educational level could be improved to high school level, 31.2% of the children could be fully immunised. Similarly in the same year if the whole country could have the same socio-economic conditions of the western Turkey 41.0% of the children could be fully immunised.

CONCLUSION

The neo-liberal economic policies in Turkey began with the military coup on September 12 1980. Since that time political, ideological and economic regulations have been introduced in order to transfer all of the public sector, including the health sector, to the market. Since that time all of the governments have worked for the same goal. The class attack of bourgeoisie was the result of WB, IMF and WHO programs prepared for similar peripheral capitalist countries.

The current government is trying to continue the commercialisation of the health sector with the support of national capital and their organisations. If the bourgeoisie and their compradors succeed in transferring the health sector to the dynamics of market; only those who have money will get health services, and only in accordance with their ability to pay.

Although they have not yet not reached their goal, we can already observe the negative effects in the form of deepened inequalities. Our results also confirm that both health and health service indicators were worsened and inequalities have deepened in Turkey.

There is an urgent need of regulations in favour of the group who suffer the inequalities. Regulation of income distribution, prevention of unemployment, and a tax on interest, unearned income and wealth should be introduced. There should be a free, equal, and accessible public health service, financed from the general budget.

We have to see this attack as a whole in all aspects of our lives, and have to organise a total class war against the bourgeoisie.

REFERENCES

1.Health Commission of the Left Assembly (2002), *Health in Socialist Turkey*, Nazim Kültürevi Kitapligi, Istanbul.(ISBN 975-8271-48-2)

2. Hamzaoglu O: Is GNP an Appropriate Indicator for the Development Level of a Country? *International Medical Journal*, 9 (4): 257-260, December 2002.

3.Hamzaoglu O, Belek I. Health Projections in the Natural Course of Capitalism. *Toplum Saglik Eczaci Dergisi*, 1(1): 37-52, 2001.

4. Kocaeli Chamber of Medicine (2004), *Transition in Health; what will bring to the community, the physicians and the health care staff?* 2nd Edition, ISNB 975-6984-63-5.

5. Hamzaoglu O: TÜSIAD-AKP-SAGLIK: Employers let the Governments' Mask Drop. *Toplum ve Hekim*, 19(4): 242-247, July-August 2004.

6. Hacettepe University Institute of Population Studies, Turkish Population and Health Survey 1978, Ankara.

7. Hacettepe University Institute of Population Studies (1984), Turkish Population and Health Survey 1983, Ankara.

8. Hacettepe University Institute of Population Studies (1989), Turkish Population and Health Survey 1988, Ankara.

9. Hacettepe University Institute of Population Studies, Demographic and Health Surveys Macro Int. Inc (1994), Turkish Population and Health Survey 1993, Ankara.

10. Hacettepe University Institute of Population Studies, (1999), Turkish Population and Health Survey 1998, Ankara.

11. Hacettepe University Institute of Population Studies, (2004), Turkish Population and Health Survey 2003, Ankara.

12. Kunst A E, Mackenbach J P., Measuring Socioeconomic Inequalities in Health, EUR/ICP/RPD 416, WHO, Copenhagen-28, (1994).

United Kingdom: England's health care pays high price for market reforms

John Lister

In the spring of 2005 a few snapshot views illustrate the extent of the crisis that is gripping the NHS in Britain – or more especially in England – as a result of more than two decades of largely market-based reforms.

■ In NW London, the modern Ravenscourt Park Treatment Centre, an NHS-run state of the art unit designed to fast-track elective operations, is currently standing half-empty, with losses of more than £12m a year, and facing the threat of closure or transfer to the private sector. While Ravenscourt Park only gets paid per case, the NHS patients that were expected to be referred here have instead been dispatched to rival private sector treatment centres, under contracts centrally negotiated by the government, under which the NHS pays the full cost regardless of how few or how many patients are actually treated.

■ In SW London, Kingston (a busy District General Hospital) had its NHS MRI scanner standing idle throughout much of March after the budget ran out for all but urgent cases and private patients: but down the road a new private sector scanner opened up taking the least complex cases, funded by the NHS on guaranteed profits, leaving the more specialist cases to queue for NHS care.

■ In Yorkshire to the north of the country, Bradford Hospitals became the first "Foundation Trust" to fall into financial crisis, with trouble-shooters flying in from the USA to confront an £11m deficit.

■ In the midlands (Worcestershire) and elsewhere, new hospitals funded through the Private Finance Initiative (PFI) have been struggling with chronic cash problems, saddled with high overhead costs and inadequate capacity. London's first PFI hospital, the £120m Queen Elizabeth in Greenwich, has wards closed and staff laid off to balance the books because the Trust which runs the hospital now only has control of clinical budgets: all non-clinical services are part of the legally-binding contract with the private consortium that built and owns the hospital.

The situation of PFI hospitals will worsen next year with the full roll-out of a new system of "payment by results", which will pay hospital Trusts only for the actual levels of treatment delivered, on a fixed tariff of prices determined by the government. PFI hospitals, with too few beds and high, fixed, costs are at a double disadvantage in this new competitive market.

■ Within days of the May 5 General Election the first cuts in hospital services began to hit the headlines locally and nationally: Lewisham Hospital in SE London was the first to reveal an £8.5m deficit and plans for ward closures.

Labour Ministers have insisted that the new regime is designed to improve "efficiency" by introducing "contestability" between NHS Trusts and between the NHS and the private sector. As part of this, they have also insisted that they will not step in to rescue "failing" Trusts which lose out in the new market place for health care.

Accelerating reforms since 1997

Of all the developed countries, not only in Western Europe but throughout the world, the British health care system has perhaps been the most repeatedly and thoroughly subjected to both market-driven and market-style reforms over the last 25 years or so.

The process has accelerated in England since 1997 with a rapid succession of reorganisations, structural reforms, and increasing levels of privatisation and use of private sector providers, although Wales and Scotland have been able to take advantage of devolved powers to steer in a substantially different direction, looking towards the reintegration of purchasing and providing care in Scotland, and rejecting increased hospital autonomy in Wales.

The New Labour reforms revolve perhaps more than those of the Tories around the New Public Management principle of 'steering, not rowing'. Indeed it is becoming increasingly clear that the New Labour objective is that the National Health Service will become little more than a "brand name", a centralised fund that commissions and pays for patient care, rather like the "sickness funds" of European social insurance-based systems, while NHS hospitals compete on ever less favourable terms with private sector companies for a share of the budget and for the staff they need to sustain basic services.

Like the Tory reforms, the market-style policies introduced since 1997 have been strongly criticised both by doctors and by health unions for their negative impact on equity of access and treatment – while New Labour ministers argue that the reforms are necessary precisely to secure these objectives.

While the underlying principle of a public-sector, tax-funded service has been generally upheld, and the New Labour reforms have been accompanied by a substantial increase in government spending on health, partly funded through tax increases, the British reforms are in general on the most radical end of the European spectrum.

Labour ministers seeking vindication point to the sharp reduction in waiting lists and waiting times that have been achieved across much of the NHS: but the most fundamental reason for this increase in volume and pace of treatment has been the increased spending and increased numbers of front-line staff (nurses, doctors and support staff). Staff productivity has increased, while overhead costs of goods and services bought in from the private sector have spiralled upwards. A report by the Office of National Statistics in 2004 revealed that between 1995-2003 – a period in which the NHS workforce, according to the ONS, increased by 22% – spending on labour went up just 44% (from £22 billion to £32 bn).

By contrast spending on "Intermediate procurement" rose by a massive 133% – from £16 billion to £37 bn. In other words for every £1 spent on staff in 1995, just 71p was spent on goods and services from the private sector, but by 2003, for every £1 spent on staff £1.14 was spent on procurement – an increase of over 50%. Over this same period NHS output (ignoring factors which might be argued as improving the quality of care) increased by 28% according to the ONS.

New Labour is recreating a wasteful market-style system similar, if wider in scope, to the one that Thatcher began in 1989-90.

Market-driven reforms
Global budgets/Cash limits/spending cuts

In 1976, driven by an uncontrollable economic crisis and the falling value of the currency, the Labour government agreed to comply with

IMF requirements to rein in public spending, cut aspects of funding of the National Health Service, and impose for the first time global "cash limits" on health care budgets.

The incoming Thatcher government made the cash limits legally binding on health authorities in 1980.

Health care spending in Britain remained at a much lower level as a share of GDP than the EU and OECD averages throughout the 1990s, and only after 2002 did the New Labour government embark upon a conscious policy of injecting substantial above-inflation increases to the NHS budget to raise it towards the EU average.

By 2004-5 the NHS budget, at £67 billion was double the 1996-97 figure. Billions of this extra spending, however, are funnelled into contracts with private health providers, making profits for the private companies, whilst many NHS hospitals are facing bigger than ever cash deficits and are being forced to close beds and cut jobs.

Rationalisation

The market-driven squeeze on health spending was tightened in the mid 1980s by explicit cutbacks which created successive years of zero or negative growth in NHS spending, and prompted crisis measures by health authorities – a fresh round of rationalisation of service provision, including hospital closures.

Waiting lists for treatment grew rapidly during the 1980s, and it was the resulting prevalence of delays even for the treatment of urgent cancers and child heart operations in the winter of 1987-88 which generated the political imperative for Thatcher's review of the NHS.

The rapid rundown in numbers of acute hospital beds which characterised the 1980s and early 1990s – driven by the expansion of day surgery and new anaesthetics and surgical techniques – has largely come to a halt, and government guidance has underlined the need for additional hospital and "intermediate" capacity to deal with a rising proportion of older patients.

However the very heavy cutbacks in beds for older patients and mental health beds have continued, although at a slower pace than the early 1990s.

While the main drive to closure of acute beds has weakened, and while in theory all new hospital schemes should now contain at least as many beds as the facilities they replace, many plans for costly new hospitals to be funded through the Private Finance Initiative are again raising the issue of reducing numbers of acute hospital beds to hold down the size (and cost) of the project: recent examples include schemes in Epsom & St Helier (SW London), Birmingham, and Leicester.

New models of care

Attempts to switch to a "primary care-led NHS" in the early 1990s – with questionable levels of success –appear to be undergoing a revival. New schemes seek to restrict the size of new costly hospital projects by switching services from hospital to primary care.

Market-style reforms
Decentralisation

Increased hospital autonomy began with the establishment of "self-governing" provider units as NHS Trusts as part of the Conservative government's market-style reforms in the 1990s.

This was not initially accompanied by increased independence for the purchasing health authorities, which remained centrally accountable through regional health authorities to the Department of Health, which also controlled all key lay appointments to health authorities and Trust boards.

More recent reorganisations in England have scrapped regional health authorities and established 28 Strategic Health Authorities, and replaced Primary Care Groups with Primary Care Trusts (PCTs), local commissioning bodies which within a few years were expected to control upwards of 80% of the total NHS budget for primary, community and hospital services.

The early promise that PCTs would exercise substantial local autonomy has been thrown into question by the Department of Health's insistence that PCTs in Oxfordshire had no choice but to agree to the establishment of a controversial private sector Treatment Centre delivering cataract treatment, despite PCT concerns that it would undermine the financial viability of Oxford's existing NHS Eye Hospital.

The widely-held view that PCTs have failed adequately to establish themselves as effective purchasing bodies forcing maximum value from hospital Trusts has led to fears among some observers that these organisations, established in 2002, will in turn be reorganised and merged into new, larger and less accountable bodies after the 2005 election.

One strongly critical BMJ Editorial on the issue notes that:

"Reorganisations are a clumsy reform tool, and research shows that they seldom deliver the promised benefits.

Every reorganisation produces a transient drop in performance, and it takes a new organisation at least two or three
years to become established and start to perform as well as
its predecessor. Yet the NHS is reorganised every two years
or so, which probably means it sees all the costs of each
reorganisation and few of the benefits."

Purchaser/provider split and contracts

The Conservatives' market-style reforms were implemented from the
spring of 1991. The government had rejected many of the stock proposals of the radical right, for voucher-style schemes and other mechanisms
to privatise the delivery of more health care, and for the imposition of
fees and charges for treatment or for "hotel services".

Instead the plans had been built around the concept of creating an
'internal market', which would drive up efficiency and quality through
competition between rival providers. The kernel of the reforms was the
separation of the secondary care sector, which had for 40 years been
planned and run by local health authorities, into purchasers (remodelled
and smaller health authorities, spending budgets allocated by central
government on the basis of the age profile of the local catchment population) and providers –'self-governing' NHS Trusts.

A further key factor in the dynamics of this new 'market' was to be
the encouragement of the larger, group practices of GPs – who had
always been independent, self-employed contractors rather than NHS
employees – to see themselves and the services they delivered as a business, by becoming "fund-holding" practices.

Fund-holders would receive an annual cash-limited budget based on
the demographic profile of their list of patients, from which they would
purchase non-emergency inpatient and outpatient care from hospitals.

They were encouraged to use this new bargaining power to "shop
around" for low prices, and high quality services for their patients
(quality in many cases being linked to reduced waiting times). Fund-
holders would be free to refer patients to any Trust, while those smaller
practices and GPs who elected not to become fund-holders would be
restricted to those Trusts where their local health authority had negotiated a contract. As an additional incentive to join the scheme, fund
holders were given a very generous calculation of their cash allocation,
and were to be permitted to retain any unspent surplus in their budgets
for patient care at the end of each year. Some began to accrue very substantial amounts.

GPs were urged to opt for the autonomy of fund-holding, and the government steadily reduced the size of the practice required and found new ways of drawing in groups of GPs. By 1997 a majority of patients were covered by fund-holding practices.

Up until the election in 1997, Labour in opposition promised that it would abolish the wasteful and competitive internal market, and replace it with a duty of different sections of the NHS to work in partnership. However the 1997 White Paper The New NHS – Modern, Dependable fell well short of abolition: it retained the essential purchaser/provider split, and retained Trusts as the provider unit for secondary and specialist care: only GP fund-holding was swept away in a curious half-way house arrangement which established Primary Care Groups (PCGs), open to all GPs in every locality, which would act as a sub-committee of the district health authority.

In the event PCGs themselves were to be swiftly swept away and replaced with Primary Care Trusts, in which the role of GPs and primary care practitioners was much more marginal, and which would become the larger and less accountable bodies that still exist today through a process of mergers.

Provider autonomy

Under the Thatcher reforms, Trusts became 'public corporations', each governed by a Trust Board of directors composed of executive directors and direct and indirect government appointees, conducting most business behind closed doors. Their main income would come from contracts with purchasing health authorities, for which they would be required to compete on the basis of price and quality.

They were required to balance their books each year, to pay capital charges on the assets they take over, and to generate a 6% return each year on their assets.

Trusts were encouraged to generate income by whatever means they saw fit, including advertising and the expansion of their provision of private beds for fee-paying patients. They would be "free" to vary pay scales for their staff (effectively breaking up the national pay framework), to sell surplus property assets and use the returns, and to compete for contract revenue from local or more distant Trusts, and from fund-holding GPs.

The reforms were highly controversial – and strongly opposed both by the BMA and by the health unions. They required a system for pricing and billing for each item of service delivered to patients, and thus began a commodification of health care which could potentially have provided a base from which means-tested user fees could have been introduced. Once the first wave of Trusts had launched in 1991, the remaining hospitals and community services came under increasing pressure to seek Trust status.

Prior to this substantial restructuring, the Tory government had during the 1980s introduced early experiments foreshadowing the type of measures that later became known as "New Public Management". A new tier of general managers had been created as a result of the Griffiths Report in 1983 to replace the more traditional "administrators" and begin the process of separating out the management of provider units from the management of health authorities.

A number of these managers were brought in from industrial and other experience outside the NHS, and the restructuring can be seen as reinforcing the hand of management in relation to the professional powers of doctors, and laying the basis for subsequent market-style reforms.

There was an accompanying rhetoric promoting the idea of applying "business methods" to the NHS, which served to divert some public and media attention from the substantial increase in bureaucracy and associated costs that resulted from the reforms (numbers of admin and clerical staff rose by 18% in the decade to 1991, while admin costs rose from 6% of NHS spending to 11% over the same period.

More Provider autonomy

In the recent round of reforms, "three star" Trusts, already shown to be performing best against the government's targets and star ratings system, were urged to apply to become 'Foundation Trusts', on the model of similar hospitals in Sweden and Spain and Portugal's "hospital companies (Hospitals SA).

Foundations are non-profit public companies (or even described as 'mutuals'), controlled by local boards and accountable not to the Secretary of State but to a new Independent Regulator (known as Monitor).

Foundations have been promised new freedoms to engage in "entrepreneurial" activity over and above the freedoms available to non-foundation Trusts. However the government was forced to retreat from early promises that Foundation Trusts would be free to borrow on the money markets, and free to expand private beds and services: indeed ministers insisted that private activity and borrowing will be strictly limited in

Foundation Hospitals – though it is not clear how this would be policed by Monitor.

The legislation eventually passed through the Commons with a majority of just 17, and only a limited number of Foundations had been established before the 2005 General Election: however the Blair government made clear very early in the process that if they were re-elected then all hospitals would be pressed to become Foundations.

The exception is Wales and Scotland, where the National Assembly and the Scottish Parliament have both exercised their devolved powers and chosen not to establish foundation hospitals.

The extent of the autonomy on offer to Foundations was thrown into question in the autumn of 2004, when one of the first wave, Bradford Hospitals, found itself facing a substantial deficit (predicting a £4 million deficit after just six months) in place of the modest surplus it had predicted in its business plan.

Despite the fact that this level of deficit is modest compared with many NHS Trusts, Monitor immediately intervened, and called in a firm of New York-based business trouble-shooters to sort out the growing financial crisis. The company, Alvarez & Marsal (A&M), was chosen and called in by Monitor: but the costs of flying in the team of "turnaround management consultants" (who had to be told that British healthcare is priced in pounds and not dollars) had to be paid by the Bradford Trust.

Yet even while the regulator has seen fit to intervene so publicly and dramatically, Ministers predictably washed their hands of the whole business. In the House of Commons Health Secretary John Reid has issued a statement refusing to answer parliamentary questions on any foundation trusts, declaring that:

> "Ministers are no longer in a position to comment on, or provide information about, the detail of operational management within such Trusts. Any such questions will be referred to the relevant Trust chairman."

Provider payment reform

The internal market reforms of 1991 introduced the notion of annual contracts drawn up between health authority purchasers and providers, which would be monitored to ensure compliance: additional cases above a certain threshold would incur additional payments, while under-performing Trusts could face a loss of revenue.

However throughout the 1990s most negotiations and most treatment took place on the basis of block contracts, with only GP fund-holders, with much smaller numbers of patients, seeking special treatment for individual cases: prices varied widely from Trust to Trust depending on the cost pressures faced by the hospital, and sometimes the skill mix of the staff and the way in which the cost of each treatment was calculated.

However as part of its new, wider-reaching marketising reform, New Labour has moved to introduce a much more complex system of "payment by results" (PBR), to be phased in for providers from April 2004.

This will mean that NHS Trusts will be paid on a fixed scale of "reference costs" for each item of treatment they deliver – the old system of block contracts will be scrapped.

The new structure seems designed to create a new framework within which Foundation Trusts can secure a wider share of the available contract revenue in a competitive health "market", while Trusts less well resourced, or whose costs for whatever reason are higher than the reference price, could lose out.

However it is also the case that by effectively commodifying health care at such a basic level, the PBR system facilitates the New Labour objective of breaking down the barriers between the public and private sectors, and making much greater use of private sector providers.

NHS Trusts therefore have increasingly to compete not only against other NHS Trusts, but also against private hospitals which have a much more selective, purely elective, and thus much less complex and costly caseload.

And the pace of this competition has been forced by putting the responsibility not on to Primary Care Trusts, but on to individual patients, who will be offered a progressively wider "choice" of where they want to have their treatment – at first to include at least one private hospital. By the end of 2005 Primary Care Trusts will be obliged to offer almost all patients a "choice" of providers – including at least one private hospital – from the time they are first referred but eventually (from 2008) any patient will be allowed to choose any hospital which can deliver treatment at the NHS reference cost.

Irrespective of what patients may choose, ministers have made clear that they want at least 10% of NHS elective operations to be carried out by the private sector in 2006, rising to 15% by 2008.

This policy has been strongly criticised, not least by the BMA, but also by studies produced by London NHS managers for Health

Secretary John Reid, which warned that the plans were "problematic, unaffordable" and of "no benefit" in London, since they would have serious impact on the financial stability and viability of NHS Trusts. The Commons Public Accounts Committee has warned that the policy could result in private sector providers "cream skimming" the most straightforward and lucrative cases, leaving NHS hospitals with reduced resources to cope with the chronic, the complex and the costly patients: it could also give GPs perverse incentives to refer patients to hospitals which did not have adequate facilities or medical support.

There has been growing concern that hospitals which lose out as patients choose to go elsewhere could be forced to close departments – or close down altogether: ministers and senior NHS officials have said that they are willing to see this happen, arguing that it would not be their policy, but patients who made the decision. However it is not only this factor that could push hospitals into difficulties, but also the problems faced by hospitals where for whatever reason operations are currently costing above the NHS reference cost, which will face a substantial cut in revenue under PBR.

Even where hospitals have been charging less than the new reference cost, and would stand to make windfall gains under the new system, the Primary Care Trusts which buy services from them would find their budgets cut. Estimates of the mis-match in funding are as high as £1 billion a year across the NHS, with some Trusts set to lose very heavily.

This new market-style system makes no reference to social and other inequalities, and runs the risk of funnelling an ever-larger share of the NHS budget to the best-resourced and largest Trusts and GP practices at the expense of those struggling to cope in more deprived areas.

But the new system also represents the end of 30 years of efforts to equalise allocations of NHS spending on the basis of population and local health needs.

Now PCTs in areas where Trusts are currently delivering services below the new NHS reference costs will require extra cash to pay an increased fee – which will become a "surplus" for the Trust. Conversely PCTs whose Trusts currently deliver relatively high-cost treatment will see their cash allocations reduced.

None of this bears any relation to social deprivation, the age profile or relative health of the population: the new market system emerges as the enemy of equality.

The prospect of widespread financial instability has forced a delay and a phased introduction of the new payment system, which was to have applied to 70% of treatments by April 2005, but in the run-up to the General Election has already been postponed by 12 months, and may well be postponed further.

Purchase services from private sector

New Labour's commitment to buying an increasing volume of NHS treatment from the private sector began with the signing of a Concordat with the private sector hospitals in 2000, and, more recently, the signing of contracts for the establishment of a new network of privately-run for-profit Treatment Centres that will deliver certain types of elective care to NHS patients.

The government is determined to forge ahead regardless of the mounting evidence that many of the private units are neither needed nor welcome. The case of the private treatment centre specialising in cataract operations, to be foisted upon Oxfordshire's Primary Care Trusts despite the evidence that it will cut the ground from below the well-established Oxford Eye Hospital has achieved national notoriety.

Early in 2005 the government invited private tenders to deliver a further 250,000 operations a year, worth an estimated £500 million annually: in addition another £400m worth of X-rays, scans, blood tests and pathology tests will be hived off to the private sector.

These moves will almost double the number of private sector operations to be purchased by the NHS, pushing the government's total spend in the "independent sector" up towards £1.5 billion – two thirds of the total £2.3 billion turnover of the private medical industry in 2003.

Among the companies hoping to cash in on this new bias in favour of privatisation are Swedish private health firm Capio and Nuffield Hospitals.

It is clear that in some areas, especially those where private hospitals are few and far between, PCTs could find themselves obliged to meet their targets for increased private sector referrals by effectively denying patients the option of NHS care.

Critics are also warning that if large numbers of individuals are encouraged to opt for a private sector provider, they could trigger the financial collapse and even closure of local health services or even whole NHS hospitals – even those which are doing well under the current system.

Hospitals which lose a slice of their elective care will see their unit costs go up, as existing capacity is used by fewer patients, and as they are left to deal with the cases which the private sector does not wish to treat.

The BMA has warned that even where some lose hospitals less than 10 percent of their patients to private sector or other NHS Trusts the effects could force them to close.

Even where public capital has already been invested in state of the art NHS-run treatment centres there is no long-term guarantee that these will remain viable or operational. Some are already in trouble.

The blatant bias that is being shown in favour of private providers and against the NHS is exposed by the problems faced by one of the pioneering NHS-run treatment centres, the Ambulatory Care and Diagnostic (ACAD) unit at Central Middlesex Hospital. While the privately-run treatment centres receive long-term guaranteed income on a "play or pay" basis, and have up to now been allowed to charge higher than NHS reference costs, none of these conditions applies to NHS treatment centres.

Elsewhere NHS consultants have been instructed by managers to pass over a share of their waiting list workload for treatment in private sector units – but no such pressure exists to maintain the flow of patients to NHS units.

By the winter of 2004 ACAD, like other NHS treatment centres, reported having spare capacity to treat thousands more patients: instead partly-used NHS facilities result in rising costs and poor productivity – giving ministers a ready-made pretext for favouring an apparently cheaper and more efficient private sector.

University College London Hospital (UCLH) has warned that it may have to scale down its treatment centres if the odds remain stacked against them: but it seems that the government's fixation with expanding the private hospital sector could lead them to ban Foundation Trusts like UCLH from bidding for the provision of the next round of treatment centres in the January tendering process. Ministers want to take every opportunity to convince private firms of the government's commitment to privatising an ever-increasing share of clinical care.

An underlying difficulty for those arguing in favour of a greater 'partnership' between the public and private medical sectors is the chronic and worsening shortage of suitably skilled professional staff, all of whom in Britain are trained by the NHS. The relatively small scale of private medicine and the long-standing under-occupancy of private hospital beds has meant that any additional caseload diverted from the NHS to private hospitals must result in intensified competition to recruit and retain nursing and medical staff.

Competition

Although competition on the basis of price has now been ruled out, with the phased introduction of Department of Health reference prices for specific treatments, competition for contracts seems set to be fiercer than ever once the PBR system is phased in.

Ministers appear to be set on a course of building up sufficient capacity in the private sector to generate a real fear that failing NHS Trusts will be allowed close down, with services delivered from alternative private providers. What this scenario does not address is the wide range of emergency and other services which are currently available only from NHS hospitals, and which the private sector has shown no interest in providing.

Privatisation

During the last two decades the UK has been characterised by the World Bank as one of the world's most active privatising governments, although in health care this has largely centred on non-clinical services.

From 1984 onwards hospitals were required to put their main ancillary services (catering, cleaning and laundry – later followed by portering and security services) out to competitive tender, with evidence of mounting government pressure to accept the lowest tender regardless of quality.

Even where this did not result in the outright privatisation of services, this early exercise in "steering, not rowing" served to introduce the notion of partial private provision within a publicly-funded service, separated off these "hotel" services from the clinical services in each hospital, and resulted in a large scale reduction in jobs, pay and conditions for the lowest-paid staff, with questionable effects on levels of hygiene, patient care and staff morale.

The first wave of PFI hospitals were delivered on contracts which included the privatisation of the core non-clinical support services: subsequent PFI schemes incorporate the privatisation of the management of these services, with support staff seconded to the private contractor – a system which has yet to demonstrate any evidence of success in the improvement of quality or efficiency.

User fees

The rapid, above-inflation rises in prescription charges which characterised the period of Conservative rule from 1979 have ended, but prescriptions for the 20% or so of patients who are not exempt have continued to increase with inflation. No additional user fees have been imposed: the NHS remains largely free at point of use.

In Wales, the National Assembly has made use of its autonomous powers to freeze, reduce and eventually eliminate prescription charges, which generate little revenue but serve to deter the working poor from fully accessing the treatment they require.

Steps to control medical professionals

A dimension of many of the reforms since 1990 has been the attempt by successive governments to control the cost and quality of services delivered by hospital consultants and by GPs. Conservative reforms attempted to discipline consultants by incorporating them as directors of departments that would be obliged to work to fixed budgets.

Those who opted to become GP fundholders from 1991 were the first primary care doctors to be subjected to the discipline of cash limits: this regime has now been extended by the New Labour government to cover the whole of the NHS. Since 2000, a succession of new contracts have been used in a bid to curb the amount of private work that can be undertaken by consultants, and stipulate a minimum number of hours that must be worked for the NHS, while a new GP contract has also stipulated new tasks and duties.

Patient choice

As discussed above, a key factor driving a new round of market competition and also drawing more NHS spending into the private sector is the new system of 'patient choice', which began with a scheme under which patients waiting six months or more for treatment were entitled to transfer to another NHS – or private sector – provider.

Health Secretary John Reid now insists that patient choice is a more fundamental principle than maintaining local access to NHS hospital services, following a line from Tony Blair in October 2003:

"Choice is not a betrayal of our principles.

"It is our principles".

PFI/PPP

Ironically the payment by results system will cause the biggest problems for new hospitals funded under the Private Finance Initiative (PFI) – which are saddled with high, fixed overhead costs for non-clinical services, in the form of legally-binding, index-linked payments to the PFI consortium, while lacking spare beds and capacity to take on additional patients. Since the non-clinical costs are largely fixed and non-negotiable, the only area of activity capable of variation is clinical care – resulting in the £120m Queen Elizabeth Hospital in Woolwich running with wards closed to save on staffing costs.

The attempts by the Tory government to privatise the provision of capital for major hospital development projects through the private finance initiative (PFI) was a part of their market-style reform of health care. Although the policy was introduced from 1992, alongside year-by-year reduction of allocations of NHS capital, but the concerns of private sector companies that their investment may not be secure in the context of Trusts struggling for financial viability meant that the Conservatives were unable to finalise any PFI schemes, and no new hospitals were built under PFI until the New Labour government legislated new guarantees for private consortia after 1997.

By spring 2004, 21 new hospitals, capital value £1.5 billion, were complete and operational, with 10 more new hospitals, capital value £1.9 billion under construction. A further three new hospitals, total value £1.7 billion, were still in negotiation, with more lining up for approval. Nine tenths of all new hospital projects were being funded through PFI, with only one major hospital funded through capital from the Treasury.

More PFI hospital projects, worth £4 billion, were given the go-ahead by John Reid during the summer of 2004, many of them reflecting the massive cost inflation of PFI schemes since the first wave was rubber-stamped back in 1998.

While the average cost of a new hospital project in the first wave PFI was £75m, there are now a series of schemes under consideration costing over £500m, raising serious questions of affordability and value for money.

Despite the soaring costs and less than satisfactory performance of many of the PFI hospitals, most of which are already mired in debt long before PBR is implemented, there has been little attempt at ministerial or Department level to learn from the failures in the design and build quality of the first wave of PFI hospitals, many of which proved difficult and uncomfortable places for staff and patients alike.

More detailed critiques of the theory and practical experience of PFI as a method for financing health care facilities have been set out elsewhere (Lister 2001, Pollock 2004): but the government's commitment to establish upwards of £7 billion of privately-owned facilities to be leased by the NHS is equivalent to the privatisation of a third of the NHS property asset base when New Labour took office. PFI-built hospitals and other assets are themselves now being traded as risk-free profit-streams in the financial markets.

Vulnerable: but not a priority

This outline has not had the scope to include a discussion of the very substantial privatisation of long-term care of the elderly which has taken place in the last 25 years, resulting in the closure of more than half the NHS provision of elderly care beds and a proliferation of for-profit nursing homes.

Nor is it possible in this overview article to explore the real and growing problems in resourcing and funding mental health services, as the old-style hospital in-patient services continue their rapid reduction, but the renewed cash squeeze serves to limit the necessary expansion of community-based services to take their place.

In each case the specialist care for these potentially vulnerable groups of patients has been significantly omitted from the government's lists of targets and priorities for NHS Trusts and PCT commissioners: so as the cash pressures weigh down on the NHS, these services are seen as "soft" and easy targets for cuts, with relatively little media focus and few active campaigns to pus them into public view.

The harsh regime of a market system – which pits a comprehensive public health care system into unfair competition with selective and purely elective services delivered by a protected, government-sponsored, profit-seeking private sector – makes it more likely that gaps in care and social inequality will widen, as commissioners, managers and ministers collectively blame "patient choice" for the financial failure of hard-pressed local hospitals.

Blair has made clear that he wants his third and final term as Prime Minister to leave an irreversible 'legacy', in the form of reform in health and education. Campaigners, including the health unions which continue to fund New Labour's election effort, will be struggling to stop Blair, like a victorious hunter of old, mounting the stuffed and mounted head of a slaughtered NHS as a trophy on his wall after he steps down.

Much of the above text is an adapted version of the section on the UK in the book *Health Policy Reform: Driving the Wrong Way?* by John Lister, published July 2005 and reprinted July 2007 by Middlesex University Press www.mupress.co.uk

References

Bach S (2000) 'Decentralisation and privatisation of municipal services: the case of health services', Sectoral activities programme Working Paper ILO, Geneva, November 2000.

Busse R, van der Grinten T and Svensson PG (2002) 'Regulating entrepreneurial behaviour in hospitals: theory and practice', in Saltman et al (2002)

Caldwell K, Francome C and Lister J (1998) *The Envy of the World*. NHS Support Federation, London

Carvel J (2004) 'NHS Trusts bullied into private contracts: Chairman lost job for resisting cataracts deal with foreign firm', *The Guardian* 1 June

CMMH (Central Manchester and Manchester Children's University Hospitals NHS Trust) (2003) Outline agreement of the Trust, Manchester Primary Care Trusts, the Strategic Health Authority, Private Finance Unit and the Review team. Nov 14, http://www.cmmc.nhs.uk/your_trust/trustboard/dec2003/agenda_item8.pdf, accessed 29.5.04

Conrad M (2005) 'Expert warns of more delays on PBR rollout', *Public Finance* March 18-24:8

Coombes R (2005) 'Private providers must be stopped from skimming off easy cases', *British Medical Journal* 330:691

DoH (Department of Health) (2000a) *National Beds Inquiry*. February 10, HMSO, London

DoH (Department of Health) (2000b) *Shaping the future NHS: long-term planning for hospitals and related services*. Consultation document on the findings of the National Beds Inquiry. HMSO, London

DoH (Department of Health) (2002a) *Growing capacity: Independent Sector Diagnosis and Treatment Centres*. HMSO, London

DoH (Department of Health) (2002b) 'New generation surgery-centres to carry out thousands more NHS operations every year', Press release 2002/00529 December 23, HMSO, London

Gould M (2005) 'Managers move to quell protest over bed cuts', *Health Service Journal* March 24:8

Guichard S (2004) 'The reform of the health care system in Portugal', Economics Department Working Papers No. 405, October, OECD, Paris

Ham C (1999) *Health Policy in Britain*. (4th edition) Macmillan, London

Hart J Tudor (1994) *Feasible Socialism – The National Health Service past present and future*. Socialist Health Association, London

Hirst J (2005) 'Shock and awe', *Public Finance* (Leader) March 11-17:2

Knight R (2004) 'Consumer group attacks "illusion of choice" in public services', *Financial Times* December 1

Lister J (2003a) *SW London Hospitals Under Pressure*. Battersea & Wandsworth TUC, London

Lister J (2003b) *The PFI Experience, Voices from the frontline*. UNISON, London

Lister J (2003c) *Not So Great: voices from the frontline at Swindon's Great Western*

Hospital. UNISON, London

Lister J (2004) Beds and jobs axed as Trusts cut back, *Health Emergency* No. 60, December 2004.

Lister J (2004) *Gambling with our lives: a response to the consultation document from Merton, Sutton and Mid Surrey NHS.* October, UNISON Epsom & St Helier Branch, St Helier Hospital

Mayo E and Lea R (2002) *The Mutual Health Service.* November, New Economic Foundation, London

McGauran A (2004) 'Moving 15% of procedures to private sector will wreck NHS', *British Medical Journal* 329:1257

Mossialos E and Mrazek M (2002) 'Entrepreneurial behaviour in pharmaceutical markets and the effects of regulation', in Saltman et al (2002)

Paterson R and Walker M (1997) *A very peculiar practice: the case against GP fundholding.* April, UNISON /NHS Support Federation, London

Pollock AM (2004) *NHS plc The privatisation of our health care.* Verso, London

Pollock AM and Price D (2003) *In Place of Bevan? Briefing on the Health and Social Care (Community health and standards) Bill 2003.* September, Catalyst, London

Rivett G (1998) *From Cradle to Grave.* Kings Fund, London

Saltman RB, Busse R and Mossialos E (eds) (2002) Regulating entrepreneurial behaviour in European health care systems, Open University Press, Buckingham

Smith P (2003) 'We might not save flops, judges Dredge', *Health Service Journal* 25 September: 6-7

Smith R (2005) 'NHS at war', *Evening Standard* 18 January, www.thisislondon.co.uk/til/jsp/modules/Article/print.jsp?itemId=15987842, accessed 24.01.05

Timmins N (2004) 'Health service revolution dogged by controversy', *Financial Times* January 13

Timmins N (2004) 'Shunned hospitals "may go bust" as patients get choice', *Financial Times* November 23:4

Timmins N (2005) 'NHS Trusts hit financial trouble despite cash injection', *Financial Times* January 5

Walshe K, Smith J, Dixon J, Edwards N, Hunter DJ, Mays N, Normand C and Robinson R (2004) 'Primary care trusts: premature reorganisation, with mergers, may be harmful', *British Medical Journal* Editorial 329:871-872.

Ward S (2005) ' "Limit growth" on private care in NHS', *Public Finance* March 11-17:8

Whitfield D (1992) *The Welfare State.* Pluto, London

A REVIEW OF DATA ON THE U.S. HEALTH SECTOR

Nicholas Skala and Ida Hellander

This report presents information on the state of the U.S. health sector in late summer 2005. It includes data on the uninsured and underinsured and their access to health care, on socioeconomic inequalities in health care, and on the rising costs of health insurance. It also presents information on the role of corporate money in health and health care, focusing on the pharmaceutical and hospital industries. The authors include an update on Medicare HMOs and the prescription drug bill, the results of some recent public opinion polls on health care, and some international comparisons of health systems. The article ends with recent data on health (medical) savings accounts and high-deductible insurance plans.

Uninsured and underinsured

The number of uninsured Americans rose to 45 million in 2003 (the most recent year for which data are available), an increase of 1.4 million from 2002. The percentage of the population without coverage increased from 15.2 percent in 2002 to 15.6 percent in 2003. The proportion of uninsured children remained at 11.4 percent in 2003, or 8.4 million kids. Approximately 2.6 million fewer Americans had employer-based health insurance coverage in 2003 than in 2002. The percentage of Americans covered by employment-based insurance declined from 61.3 percent in 2002 to 60.4 percent in 2003. The large drop in job-based coverage was masked by a 2.6 million increase in the number of people covered by government programs. Medicare coverage increased by 600,000 to 13.7 percent (U.S. Census Bureau, "Income, Poverty, and Health Insurance Coverage in the United States: 2003," August 26, 2004).

Oregon's uninsured rate in 2004 surpassed the national uninsured rate for the first time in a decade, with 17 percent of the state's population (609,000 people) lacking coverage, the highest rate since 1992. An additional 257,000 people reported they had gone without insurance at some point during the year. Oregon was touted as a leader in health reform in the 1990s for its Medicaid rationing scheme based on ranking medical services by their cost-effectiveness, but the scheme failed to keep up with the rising number of uninsured or to control rising health costs (Colburn, *Oregonian*, January 18, 2005).

In California, only about half (53.8%) of residents were covered by employment-based insurance in 2003, far below the national average of 60.4 percent, according to the UCLA (University of California, Los Angeles) Center for Health Policy. More than 6.5 million Californians are uninsured (Rojas, *Sacramento Bee*, February 7, 2005).

The proportion of children covered through a parent's employer fell from 62.3 percent in 2000 to 58.3 percent in 2003. The percentage of children covered by public programs grew from 20.9 percent to 26.4 percent during the same period. In FY 2003, SCHIP (State Children's Health Insurance Program) enrollment increased 9.0 percent, bringing total enrollment to 5.8 million children (Maher, *Wall Street Journal*, February 15, 2005).

Of all children enrolled in Medicaid or SCHIP, 27.7 percent are no longer enrolled 12 months later. Of those, 45.4 percent are dropped despite remaining eligible and having no other insurance (Sommers, *Health Services Research*, 40(1):59–78, 2005).

Disabled adults are being denied needed health care because of Medicare's two-year waiting period to receive benefits, according to a study by the Commonwealth Fund. Federal law requires that disabled individuals wait two years from the time they receive Social Security Disability Insurance (SSDI) before their Medicare takes effect. Disabled Americans under age 65 account for 6 million of Medicare's 40 million beneficiaries. One-third of the 1.2 million disabled Americans currently on the waiting list have no health insurance. In interviews with researchers, individuals on the waiting list reported forgoing needed care and feeling out of control of their own lives. Many suffer irrevocable physical and mental deterioration during the waiting period because of skipped doctor visits, treatments, and medications. Ironically, many participants who begin receiving SSDI benefits find the small cash benefit makes them ineligible for Medicaid. Some with incomes below the poverty line never meet their state's criteria for Medicaid eligibility (Bob Williams, "Waiting for Medicare: Experiences of Uninsured People with Disabilities in the Two-Year Waiting Period for Medicare," Commonwealth Fund, October 2004).

A federal judge ruled that Illinois's Medicaid program fails to provide a minimum acceptable standard of medical care to 600,000 children. Federal law requires that children covered by Medicaid receive regular vision, dental, and hearing screenings as well as immunizations and preventive services; at least 80 percent of children enrolled in Medicaid must receive at least one service each year. An independent analysis of state Medicaid claims from 1998 to 2001 showed that 43 percent of infants in the program had not received a single medical exam, and more than 75 percent of children had not received a recommended blood lead–screening test. Lawyers for the children cited physicians' refusal to treat Medicaid patients because of low reimbursement rates as the principal reason for the lack of access. U.S. District Judge Joan Lefkow dismissed the argument of the state's attorneys, who asserted that children who couldn't find a physician to treat them should have looked for a free clinic, as "sheer fantasy" (Sachdev, *Chicago Tribune*, August 25, 2004; Memisovski v. Maram (N.D. Ill.), 1203).

The proportion of large employers offering health benefits to retirees fell from about two-thirds in 1988 to about one-third in 2004. Additionally, about 79 percent of companies that still offered retiree health care coverage in 2004 increased premiums. Jonathan Gruber, a professor of economics at MIT (Massachusetts Institute of Technology), said, "In this day and age, retiree health insurance is perhaps the single biggest determinant of retirement" (Porter and Walsh, *New York Times*, February 9, 2005).

A federal judge granted a temporary injunction in February 2005 to block new rules that would allow companies to dump health care coverage for aging retirees while providing them to younger retirees. The Equal Employment Opportunity Commission planned to introduce the rule, which would allow employers to drop coverage for workers once they became eligible for Medicare, but the court found that offering two separate benefit packages would violate U.S. antidiscrimination law (Caruso, *AP/Pittsburgh Post Gazette*, February 5, 2005).

The "American Jobs Creation Act of 2004," signed into law by President Bush last fall gives large employers new options to cut retired workers' health care benefits. Previously, although large companies were allowed to withdraw surplus pension assets to pay for retiree medical costs, they were barred from making reductions in health benefits for five years after the transfer and were required to maintain the same spending amount per capita during the period. Under the newly approved legislation, the per capita maintenance requirement is eliminated, and large companies—even those that received federal tax breaks in return for a commitment to maintain retiree benefits—are allowed to cut overall benefits for all retirees. The $16 billion telecommunications giant Lucent Technologies, which in September 2004 eliminated health benefits for 10 percent of covered retirees and their dependents, was one of the most active lobbies behind the legislation (Schultz, *Wall Street Journal*, October 12, 2004; Library of Congress, United States Public Law No. 108-357).

While the U.S. labor force has increased by only 1 percent since 2003, the number of people in temporary jobs, which often do not include health benefits, has grown 9 percent to 2.4 million. The vast majority of the growth is attributable to the increasingly popular practice by employers of hiring only temporary workers, to avoid paying costly health benefits (Porter, *New York Times*, August 19, 2004).

Uninsured Not Source of Emergency Room Crowding.

A new study shows insured, middle-class Americans, not the poor, are responsible for the overwhelming majority of overcrowded emergency departments (EDs). The study used data on 50,000 adults from the nationally representative Community Tracking Study Household Survey conducted between 2000 and 2001. More than two-thirds of adults who reported ED visits had a regular source of primary care (83%), health insurance (85%), and incomes above poverty (79%). Uninsured persons were no more likely to visit an ED than were privately insured individuals.

Moreover, those without a source of primary care were 25 percent less likely to have had an emergency visit than those with a private physician. Five or more outpatient visits in one year (odds ratio (OR) 4.2005) and poor physical health (OR 2.41) were the greatest predictors of an ED visit, followed by poor mental health (OR 1.51) and change in the usual source of care (OR 1.32). "The mistaken belief that emergency departments are overcrowded by a small, disenfranchised portion of the population can lead to misguided policy decisions," said Ellen J. Weber, M.D., the study's lead author (Weber, E. J., *Annals of Emergency Medicine*, October 19, 2004).

Less than half of uninsured Americans (48%) use or are aware of a "safety net" provider in their communities. Uninsured Americans with incomes above 300 percent of poverty (the fastest growing group of uninsured) were least likely (43%) to be aware of a safety net provider. Emergency departments were cited as a "safety net" by only 8 percent of those surveyed (Center for Studying Health System Change, Issue Brief 90, November 2004).

Higher-wage workers (those earning more than $15 per hour) are more than twice as likely to have employer-based health insurance as their lower-paid counterparts earning less than $10 an hour (88% vs. 41%). High-wage workers are also much more likely to have paid sick leave (65% vs. 34%). If low-wage workers take time off from work to seek care, they lose pay. For those without sick leave, illness can easily lead to job loss and loss of job-based coverage (Commonwealth Fund/Sara R. Collins, "Wages, Health Benefits, and Workers' Health," Issue Brief, October 2004).

A study of medical discount cards found the unregulated industry rife with fraud. Card companies offer discounts with a network of providers in return for full payment by patients at the time of service. Of 27 cards advertised in the Washington, DC, area, only five could be studied, because the other 18 had nonworking telephones. Problems with the cards include misleading advertisements, high-pressure sales tactics, false provider lists or names of providers that do not actually exist, and skimpy or nonexistent discounts. With monthly fees for the cards as high as some catastrophic insurance premiums, many cardholders were fooled into thinking they were buying insurance (Kofman et al., "Medical Discount Cards: Innovation or Illusion?" Commonwealth Fund Issue Brief, March 2005).

Tennessee Gov. Phil Bredesen, elected on a promise to rescue the state's failing Medicaid program, TennCare, announced that he intends to cut costs by dropping coverage for 323,000 adults and is currently waiting for federal approval to cut prescription drug and doctor visit coverage for an additional 400,000 people. Bredesen formerly made millions as a managed care executive at HealthAmerica, an HMO management company (Connolly, *Washington Post*, January 18, 2005; *AP/Knoxville News-Sentinel*, April 11, 2005).

Since PeachCare, Georgia's state SCHIP program, became subject to new regulations designed to cut spending by $11 million annually, more than 45,000 children have lost coverage through the program. The new rules raise PeachCare's maximum monthly premium 250 percent, from $20 to $70, and impose a payment deadline, which, if missed, causes beneficiaries to lose coverage for at least three months. PeachCare serves 190,000 children (Davis and Miller, *Atlanta Journal-Constitution*,

November 8, 2004).

The waiting list for Pennsylvania's state-subsidized health insurance for low-income adults, AdultBasic, topped 100,000 last year (2003). AdultBasic, which covers some hospital care, doctor visits, and lab work (but not medications), is available for a $30 monthly premium to state residents between the ages of 19 and 64 who have been uninsured for more than 90 days and have incomes at or below the federal poverty level. The program is financed with the state's portion of the national tobacco settlement fund, which will be reduced by $12 million next year. The average wait for AdultBasic is 16 months, and about 10,000 new people apply for the program each month (*Philadelphia Inquirer*, September 17, 2004).

The Missouri legislature approved a bill in April that would eliminate Medicaid coverage for more than 27,200 beneficiaries and end the requirement that the state's Medicaid program cover dental, vision, and hospice care. Combined with expected spending reductions in the new budget, an estimated 100,000 state residents will lose health coverage in 2005.

The legislation also calls for some families in the state's CHIP program to pay monthly premiums equal to 5 percent of their annual income. Officials estimate that 23,700 children currently in the program will lose coverage because their families can't pay (Young, *St. Louis Post-Dispatch*, April 7, 2005; Wagar and Hoover, *Kansas City Star*, April 8, 2005).

New DHHS Secretary to Restructure "Medicaid."

Instead of allowing the Institute of Medicine (IOM) to appoint the members of a new congressional commission on "restructuring" Medicaid, newly appointed Department of Health and Human Services (DHHS) Secretary Michael Leavitt will appoint the entire commission himself. A group of six Republican and six Democratic senators issued a letter urging Leavitt to let the IOM appoint the commission (Rovner, Reuters wire story, May 13, 2005; Pear, *New York Times*, May 12, 2005).

While governor of Utah in 2002, Michael Leavitt obtained a federal waiver to allow Utah to cut essential benefits from its Medicaid program and use the savings to subsidize a bare-bones health plan for low-income adults. The new plan is so skimpy it covers no hospital or specialty care.

To fund the plan, the state limited mental health and substance abuse treatment coverage, charged Medicaid patients more for physician visits, and ended a program for low-income adults with serious health problems. "This [Leavitt's] approach just gave people a lot less than they needed and made other low-income people pay for it," said Cindy Mann of Georgetown University (Lueck, *Wall Street Journal*, December 17, 2004; Pear, *New York Times*, January 19, 2005).

SOCIOECONOMIC INEQUALITY

Hospital systems in Chicago rarely invest in new facilities or equipment in black and Latino neighborhoods. Chicago's nonprofit Advocate hospital chain invested nearly 800 percent more ($232.million, compared with $26 million) on significant capital improvements at its four hospitals serving predominantly white patients than at its four hospitals serving black and Latino communities. Advocate spent $14,044 per licensed bed at predominantly white hospitals, compared with $3,184 at hospitals serving minority communities (SEIU Hospital Accountability Project, "Racial Redlining in Investment at Advocate Hospitals," December 2004).

A comparison of the mortality ratio between whites and African Americans since 1960 found that the black-white gap has changed very little in the past four decades for each of the 11 age-sex groups studied. For infants and men aged 35 and older, the mortality disparity has actually worsened. If the mortality gap could be eliminated, an estimated 83,570 excess African American deaths per year could be eliminated (Satcher et al., "What If We Were Equal? A Comparison of the Black-White Mortality Gap in 1960 and 2000," *Health Affairs*, 24(2):459–464, 2005).

In 2002, non-Hispanic blacks lost about 8.5 times as many years of potential life per 100,000 population due to HIV as non-Hispanic whites (85 vs. 72 years). Non-Hispanic blacks also had significantly more years of potential life lost than whites for homicide (962 vs. 160 years), stroke (474 vs. 173 years), and diabetes (397 vs. 160 years). Non-Hispanic blacks trailed non-Hispanic whites in at least four positive health indicators: the proportion of persons under age 65 with health insurance (81% of blacks vs. 87% of whites); adults under 65 vaccinated against influenza (50% vs. 69%); women receiving prenatal care in the first trimester (75% vs. 89%); and adults 18 years or younger who participated in regular moderate physical activity (25% vs. 35%) (U.S. DHHS, Centers for Disease Control and Prevention, National Center for Health Statistics, September and November 2004).

COSTS

U.S. health spending for 2005 is projected to be $1.94 trillion, 15.6 percent of gross domestic product (GDP), $6,423 per capita (Centers for

Medicaid and Medicare Services (CMS), Office of the Actuary, www.cms.gov). Health care expenditures in 2004 were $1.8 trillion, 15.3 percent of GDP, $6,040 per capita. By 2014, health spending is expected to consume 18.7 percent of the GDP, $3.6 trillion or $11,046 per capita. Health inflation is expected to slow to 6.6 percent in 2005, from 9.0 percent in 2002, a reduction driven almost entirely by a decrease in the use of medical care due to increased out-of-pocket costs for individuals (Heffler et al., "U.S. Health Spending Projections for 2004–2014," *Health Affairs* Web Exclusive, February 23, 2005).

Medicare Part B premiums are expected to increase by 12 percent in 2006, from $78.20 to $87.70 per month. Medicare Part B covers physician services and outpatient hospital care. Seniors on modest, fixed incomes will be hardest hit by the increases (Kaiser Daily Health Policy Report, March 29, 2005).

Health insurance premiums rose 11.2 percent from 2003 to 2004, the fourth consecutive year of double-digit increases. Premium costs outpaced the economy-wide rate of inflation by 9 percent and rose five times faster than the national increase in wages (2%) over the period. The average annual cost of single coverage rose to $3,695; family coverage rose to $9,950 (J. Gabel, *Health Affairs*, September/October 2004; *New York Times*, September 10, 2004).

In 2004, workers paid an average of 28 percent of the cost of family coverage ($2,661 of the $9,950 annual cost) and 16 percent of the cost of individual coverage ($558 of the $3,695 cost). The average employee's share of family coverage has risen by more than $1,000 since 2000 (Kaiser press release, September 9, 2004; Crenshaw, *Washington Post*, September 10, 2004; Miller, *Atlanta Journal-Constitution*, September 10, 2004).

Large employers' health premium costs are expected to increase 8 percent in 2005, to an average of $7,761 per worker, while employee contributions will increase by 14 percent, to $1,610 per employee. A survey of 200 large employers found that employers are cutting benefits and shifting costs to employees to prevent even larger premium increases (Fuhrmans, *Wall Street Journal*, October 6, 2004, and November 22, 2004; *AP/Arizona Republic*, October 6, 2004).

Health insurance premiums in the Federal Employees Health Benefits Program (FEHBP), the nation's largest buyer of health insurance, will increase by an average of 7.9 percent in 2005, following five consecutive years of double-digit increases. FEHBP, which covers 8 million federal employees and retirees, offers 249 health plans, most of which are HMO plans available only in limited regions. Eighteen of the plans that FEHBP is offering in 2005 are high-deductible health plans (Barr, *Washington Post*, September 14, 2004).

GM Blames Losses on Health Costs; Plans to Eliminate 25, 000 U.S. Jobs.

General Motors' annual health spending nearly doubled between 1996 and 2005, increasing from $3 billion to $5.6 billion ($12,443 for every current or retired worker). Moreover, GM estimates it has $63 billion in liabilities for current and future retirees' health care. GM provides coverage to 1.1 million Americans, including about 200,000 current workers, and about 130,000 older people aged 60 to 64 (not yet eligible for Medicare), their most expensive group to insure. The company's Germany- and Japan-based rivals have virtually no retiree commitments, as their U.S. operations are newer, and in their base countries, worker health expenses are covered by a national health care system. The United States' most profitable automaker, Toyota, employs only 31,000 Americans. Health benefits added $1,824 to the price of each GM vehicle produced in 2003, whereas Japan's national health insurance system left competitor Toyota with a per-vehicle health cost of $186 (Peters, *New York Times*, January 20, 2005; *Wall Street Journal*, November 16, 2004; Hakim, *New York Times*, September 15, 2004).

More than 14 million Americans spent more than 25 percent of their income on health care in 2004, up from 11.6 million Americans in 2000 (Families USA, "Health Care: Are You Better off Today Than You Were Four Years Ago?" September 28, 2004).

The proportion of working-age adults with chronic conditions whose out-of-pocket medical costs (excluding insurance premiums) exceeded 5 percent of family income rose from 15 percent in 2001 to 19 percent in 2003. Among low-income, privately insured, chronically ill people, the proportion with out-of-pocket expenses exceeding 5 percent of family income increased from 28 percent in 2001 to 42 percent in 2003, reflecting shrinking benefits (Center for Studying Health System Change, Issue Brief No. 88, September 23, 2004).

Medicaid spending increased to $276 billion in 2003, up one-third from 2000. Still, Medicaid costs grew more slowly than private insurance costs. Per-enrollee Medicaid costs for acute care rose 6.9 percent between 2000 and 2003, compared with a 9 percent increase in spending on acute care among the privately insured, and a 12.6 percent increase in employer-sponsored insurance premiums. About 68 percent of Medicaid's spending growth was for acute care, while long-term care accounted for about 30 percent of the growth. Low-income children and their parents accounted for 90 percent of Medicaid's total enrollment growth of 8.4 million people between 2000 and 2003. Only 10 percent was due to increased enrollment of the elderly and disabled (Holahan, "Understanding the Recent Growth in Medicaid Spending, 2000–2003," *Health Affairs* Web Exclusive, January 26, 2005; *Health Affairs* press release, January 26, 2005).

International Brotherhood of Teamsters President James Hoffa, Jr., told the Detroit Economic Club that the United States should establish a national health care system to save companies and jobs. Hoffa called for a joint effort by companies and labor unions to develop a proposal for reform. "Rising health care costs are causing a loss of jobs and making America less competitive," he said, adding, "We need a national health care system, and we need it now" (Gallagher, *Detroit Free Press*, September 14, 2004).

States spent more on Medicaid than on elementary and secondary education combined in FY 2004. In FY 2003, Medicaid expenses accounted for an estimated 21.4 percent of total state spending, compared with 21.7 percent spent on K–12 education (National Governors' Association press release, October 12, 2004).

Taxes fund a far larger share of mental health services than does private insurance. Public spending for mental health services and substance abuse treatment in 2001 totaled $67.4 billion, compared with $36.3 billion in private spending. Public funding paid for 63 percent of mental health services and 76 percent of substance abuse treatment (Tami L. Mark et al., *Health Affairs*, March 29, 2005).

In Texas, the state legislature cut funding for mental health services under Medicaid and CHIP in 2003. Hospital emergency departments are now the only source of care for most low-income patients with mental illness in Texas. The cuts cost the state about $200 million in federal matching funds. At least 144,000 mentally ill adults lost coverage or became ineligible for services; 13,400 indigent adults and 3,400 indigent children lost coverage for medications and eligibility for therapy at community centers; 175,000 children were dropped from CHIP; and CHIP mental health benefits were halved for another 332,000 enrollees (Garrett, *Dallas Morning News*, February 7, 2005).

Small businesses are shifting costs to workers (in the form of higher-deductible coverage) or dropping coverage altogether. Sixty-three percent of small firms offered coverage in 2004, down from 68 percent in 2001. Among small employers, a whopping 31 percent offered very high-deductible ($1,000 or more) PPO (preferred provider organization) plans, compared with 6 percent of large employers (John Gabel, "Health Benefits in 2004: Four Years of Double-Digit Premium Increases Take

Their Toll on Coverage," *Health Affairs*, September/October 2004).

Businesses' retiree health benefits costs rose 12.7 percent in 2004, while retirees' share of premiums increased about 25 percent. A typical worker under the age of 65 who retired in 2004 pays $2,244 annually in premiums ($4,644 with spousal coverage). A Medicare-eligible worker who retired in 2004 pays $1,212 annually in premiums ($2,508 with spousal coverage) (Kaiser press release, December 14, 2004).

About 97 percent of all employers say the U.S. health care system is in need of significant reform (Mercer Human Resource Consulting press release, November 22, 2004).

Single-Payer Would Save California More Than $340 Billion

California would save $343.6 billion over the next ten years by implementing a single-payer system, which would slash administrative costs and allow for the bulk purchase of drugs and medical equipment, according to a study by the DC-based Lewin Group. Single-payer would provide universal coverage in California while saving about $8 billion in the first year alone. In April, state Sen. Sheila Kuehl introduced a single-payer bill (SB 840) in the state assembly. Average savings would be about $340 per California family in 2006; families making less than $150,000 annually would save between $600 and $3,000 per year. Businesses that currently offer health benefits would save 16 percent annually compared with the current system (Lawrence, *San Francisco Chronicle*, January 19, 2005).

CORPORATE MONEY AND CARE

UnitedHealth Group and Travelers Insurance paid a $20.6 million civil fine for Medicare fraud. Travelers, which formerly processed Medicare claims in six states, defrauded Medicare by more than $700 million by inflating expenditures. When UnitedHealth bought Travelers in 1995, the company continued the practice of keeping two sets of books. Hired to deliver cost savings to the program by eliminating fraud and waste by medical care providers, the companies "committed the very acts against the United States that they were hired to extirpate," the Hartford Courant said. Travelers agreed to pay the government $10.9 million; UnitedHealth Group paid $9.7 million (Levick, *Hartford Courant*, August 13, 2004).

Insurance Giants Anthem and WellPoint Merge; No Real Competition among U.S. Insurers.

Insurance giants Anthem and WellPoint are merging in an $18.4 billion deal. The new company, which will operate under the name WellPoint, will be the nation's largest insurer, with $27.1 billion in assets, 40,000 employees, and 28 million members in 13 states. California Insurance Commissioner John Garamendi was outspoken in his opposition to the deal, which lavishes $265 million in bonuses on a handful of top executives at the two firms. In return for Garamendi's approval, Anthem agreed to increase expenditures on patient care in California (it currently spends 80% of premiums on patient care, compared with an industry average of 85%) and, if executive bonuses exceed $265 million, to donate a similar amount to community health projects (Girion, *Los Angeles Times*, October 21, 2004, and November 10, 2004; Freudenheim, *New York Times*, November 10, 2004; *Wall Street Journal*, November 10, 2004).

A few insurers now control nearly every state and metropolitan market, eliminating any real competition among private health insurers. According to an American Medical Association (AMA) study, 93 percent of metropolitan areas (86 of 92) and states (25 of 27) studied are "highly concentrated" HMO markets, and 100 percent are "highly concentrated" PPO markets. The study was done before the multibillion dollar mergers of Anthem/WellPoint and UnitedHealth/ Oxford (AMA, "Competition in Health Insurance: A Study of U.S. Markets," 2004 Update, February 2005; editorial, amednews.com, April 4, 2005).

Humana bought Florida-based CarePlus Health Plans for $408 million in late 2004. CarePlus CEO Mike Fernandez personally pocketed more than $330 million from the deal, which merged South Florida's two largest Medicare HMOs (total membership, 181,000). Fernandez bought the CarePlus Medicare business along with ten clinics, a patient transportation network, and a pharmacy management company in late 2002 for $38 million (Singer, *South Florida Sun-Sentinel*, December 15, 2004).

The U.S. Supreme Court ruled that patients cannot sue their HMO for damages in state court, invalidating right-to-sue laws in ten states. A patient sued Aetna under a Texas statute that requires HMOs to "exercise ordinary care," but Aetna countersued, arguing that the 1974 Employee Retirement Security Act requires such cases to be made in federal courts where laws are more favorable to HMOs. The Supreme Court unanimously agreed with Aetna that their denials of care are "administrative decisions, not a medical determination" that could be the subject of a lawsuit. The decision effectively insulates HMOs from responsibility for delaying or denying care that injures patients, and shifts responsibility for health plan decisions to doctors (Aetna Health, Inc. v. Davila, U.S. Supreme Court Docket Number 02-1845).

A study of 8,205 patients with diabetes found that patients treated at

Veterans Administration hospitals were more likely than patients treated in HMOs to receive recommended annual blood tests (93% vs. 83%), annual eye exams (91% vs. 75%), foot exams (98% vs. 84%), and cholesterol tests (79% vs. 63%). "What this tells us is that a nationally-funded health care system can provide excellent quality of care," said lead author Eve Kerr (E. Kerr et al. *Annals of Internal Medicine*, August 17, 2004).

Medco Health Solutions, the nation's largest pharmacy benefits manager, paid more than $200 million in kickbacks to a large (unnamed) health plan in return for lucrative contracts, according to a suit filed by federal prosecutors. The allegations are part of a larger lawsuit that charges Medco with defrauding the FEHBP by switching prescriptions without physician consent, not filling prescriptions fully, and failing to inform physicians about medication interactions (Silverman, *Newark Star-Ledger*, December 2, 2004).

Mike Leavitt, the new DHHS Secretary, will retain up to $25 million in investments in his family insurance firm during his tenure in the post. The former Utah governor was head of the Leavitt Group, a firm that owns 100 insurance agencies that sell Medigap policies. Leavitt's brother, Dane, is the current president and CEO of the company (*AP/Las Vegas Sun*, December 14, 2004).

Independence Blue Cross, which administers the CHIP program in southeastern Pennsylvania, failed to inform families of their eligibility for the program. Instead, the company signed up 3,100 eligible children for its own private plan, with fewer benefits and a $45 monthly premium. The Blue Cross program covers only four physician visits (each with a $10 co-pay). CHIP covers unlimited physician office visits (without any co-pays), mental health, prescription drugs, hearing aids, eyeglasses, and routine dental care. Health advocates discovered the situation in fall 2004 while studying how Independence Blue Cross markets to low-income families and children (Uhlman, *Philadelphia Inquirer*, December 10, 2004).

Big business in California, led by McDonalds and Wal-Mart, spent $18.3 million on a ballot measure to repeal a state law that would have required large employers to provide health coverage to their employees. Despite massive spending by business, the ballot initiative succeeded by only 51 to 49 percent, a margin of 200,000 votes out of 12.6 million cast (League of Women Voters, Voter Education Fund release, Nov. 3, 2004).

Massachusetts spent more than $52 million to provide health coverage for employees of some of the state's biggest corporations in 2003 and 2004. Topping the list were Dunkin' Donuts ($3.1 million), Stop & Shop

($3 million), and Wal-Mart ($2.9 million)—each of which had more than 1,000 employees on the public coverage rolls. Typically, these low-wage workers could not afford their share of their company's health insurance premiums or were ineligible because they worked part time (Testa, Associated Press, February 1, 2005).

BIG PHARMA

Patients in the United States paid an average of 81 percent more for brand-name prescription drugs than Canada and six Western European nations in 2004, up from 60 percent more in 2000 (Sager and Socolar, Data Brief No. 7, Boston University School of Public Health, October 28, 2004).

U. S. Food and Drug Administration safety officer David Graham testified at a U.S. Senate hearing that mid-level FDA officials who warned of heart risks from Vioxx were silenced or ostracized from the agency. Graham said that warnings from the FDA drug safety office were ignored and that the FDA is "virtually incapable of protecting America" because of close ties between the agency and the pharmaceutical industry (Editorial, *Los Angeles Times*, November 23, 2004).

Graham's analysis for the FDA found that Vioxx tripled the risk of heart attack and sudden cardiac death, compared with the COX-2 inhibitor Celebrex. A 2001 study by Dr. Eric Topol, chair of the Cleveland Clinic's department of cardiovascular medicine, found that Vioxx increased heart attacks fivefold compared with naproxen (Topol, *New York Times*, October 2, 2004).

One-third of the members of the FDA panel that convened in February 2005 to determine whether to continue the sale of COX-2 inhibitors had strong ties to the drug industry. Those with ties to drug makers voted 9-1 to allow Bextra to remain on the market, and 9-1 to allow Vioxx to return to the market. In their absence, the committee would have voted both to withdraw Bextra and keep Vioxx off the market (Harris and Berenson, *New York Times*, February 25, 2005).

Drug Industry Lobbying Tops $100 Million.

The drug industry spent a record $108.6 million on federal lobbying activities in the 2004 election cycle. They retained a total of 824 lobbyists—1.5 for every member of Congress. The Pharmaceutical Research and Manufacturers of America (PhRMA), which represents more than 40 drug companies, spent $16 million on lobbying, and hired 136 lobbyists of their own. Among those lobbying on behalf of the drug and managed care industries are 30 ex-senators and ex-representatives. Drug industry employees donated $11.5 million to politicians during the 2004 election cycle, with more than two-thirds going to Republicans (Public Citizen press release, June 23, 2004; Theimer, *Las Vegas Sun*, September 1, 2004). Big Pharma is thought by some to be behind a new right-wing seniors' lobbying group. The United Seniors Association, also known as USA Next, has fashioned itself as a conservative version of the AARP (American Association of Retired Persons), advocating tax cuts, health savings accounts, and the privatization of Social Security. In 2003, the group received $24.8 million from a single source whose name was blacked out on tax records, leaving only the first letter, "P." A $20.1 million donation in 2002 was similarly blacked out. Records obtained by Public Citizen show that both PhRMA and Pfizer have been major donors to the group in past years (Tackett, *Chicago Tribune*, April 10, 2005).

A Pfizer executive, Dr. Peter Rost, broke ranks with the industry and encouraged the U.S. Congress to legalize the reimportation of prescription drugs. Rost, who directs marketing for Pfizer's growth hormone Genotropin, was formerly responsible for marketing drugs in a four-nation region of northern Europe. He noted that no pharmaceutical company or government agency warned that imported drugs were unsafe during his tenure overseas (Pear, *New York Times*, September 24, 2004).

The Florida legislature terminated a Medicaid disease management program with Pfizer after a government audit showed few savings. The Pfizer program— which exempted the giant drug firm from state-mandated discounts in the Medicaid program—was supposed to save Florida $56.3 million, but actual savings amounted to only $7.6 million. An earlier report had found that simply canceling the exemptions received by drug companies in state disease-management contracts would have saved $64.2 million (Agovino, *AP/Tallahassee Democrat*, July 27, 2004).

Individuals harmed by FDA-approved drugs would be prohibited from receiving damage awards over $250,000, regardless of the magnitude of the damage, under a proposed law (HR 534). The law would effectively end all lawsuits against drug manufacturers, despite the fact that several harmful drugs have been pulled from the market only after legal action against manufacturers exposed serious problems (Library of Congress, HR 534, February 2, 2005).

The Illinois attorney general filed suit in February against 48 pharmaceutical companies for defrauding the state and consumers by overcharging for prescription drugs. The suit cites one example in which Pharmacia—now part of Pfizer—reported an inflated wholesale price (used to calculate reimbursement rates) of $241 per month for its breast cancer drug Adriamycin, but actually charged other payers as little as $33. Attorneys in at least 19 other states have filed similar suits over the past two years. Congressional investigators estimate similar overpricing schemes have resulted in annual overpayments of at least $800 million by public health programs and $200 million by consumers (Chase and Japsen, *Chicago Tribune*, February 8, 2005).

HOSPITALS, INC.

Tenet, the nation's second-largest investor-owned hospital chain, is selling three Massachusetts hospitals to Vanguard Health Systems for $167 million. The hospitals (in Worcester, Natick, and Framingham) have been sold three times in eight years (*Boston Globe*, October 13, 2004).

The number of hospitals involved in mergers increased 136 percent, from 55 in 2003 to 130 in 2004, the largest number of hospitals undergoing mergers since 2000. The dollar value of mergers and acquisitions nearly quadrupled over the same time period, rising from $2.3 billion in 2003 to $9.1 billion in 2004 (Japsen, *Chicago Tribune*, February 10, 2005).

The Federal Trade Commission (FTC) filed a rare suit to undo a hospital merger in Illinois. The FTC is seeking to dissolve the merger of Illinois's Highland Park Hospital with the nonprofit hospital system Evanston Northwestern Healthcare. The FTC suit alleges that Evanston Northwestern used its post-merger market power to impose price increases averaging 40 to 60 percent, and up to 190 percent in at least one case, on insurers (Wysocki, *Wall Street Journal*, January 17, 2005).

THE FINAL FRONTIER: MEDICARE HMOs

Medicare HMOs are paid an average of 108 percent of what it would cost to care for their (on average healthier) enrollees under traditional Medicare. Payments run as high as 116 percent of traditional Medicare in urban areas and 123 percent in rural counties. Despite the already significant overpayments, Medicare Advantage plans are getting $10 billion in special bonus payments that the Medicare drug law set aside as an incentive for HMOs to participate in the program. Enrollment in Medicare HMOs dropped from 7 million in 1999 to 5.3 million by the end of 2003. Following a mandate to adjust payments based on enrollees' health status starting in 1999, plans that had previously profited by enrolling healthier beneficiaries began to dump seniors or slash benefits such as drug coverage. Increasing enrollment in Medicare HMOs is a top priority for DHHS Secretary Leavitt (Berenson, *Health Affairs* Web Exclusive, December 15, 2004; Pear, *New York Times*, September 17, 2004).

Medicare HMOs that dropped coverage for all but generic drugs in 2002 saved an average of $11 per member, but out-of-pocket costs to enrollees rose $16.60. Hospital admissions among beneficiaries who lost drug coverage rose by 0.3 percent (an additional 3,600 hospitalizations for the 1.2 million Medicare HMO members with generic-only coverage), while admissions declined slightly for those who kept their drug benefits. In 2002, 26 percent of Medicare HMOs covered generic medications only—three times the rate in 2001 (Christian Herman, "Effects of Generic Only Drug Coverage in a Medicare HMO," *Health Affairs* Web Exclusive, September 29, 2004).

MEDICARE DRUG BILL

Medicare's chief actuary estimates that the Medicare drug benefit will cost $1.2 trillion over the next decade. CMS administrator Mark McClellan said that figure does not account for premiums paid by beneficiaries or savings from "eliminating federal matching funds for individuals eligible for both Medicare and Medicaid."

Assuming seniors pay whopping premiums and states absorb more cuts to their already deficit-ridden Medicaid programs, the federal share of the bill's cost will be $720 billion. The Bush administration presented Congress with an original estimate of $400 billion, despite the actuary's initial estimate that the program would cost $534 billion, a figure that was not released until after the bill passed (Sherman, AP, and Pear, *New York Times*, February 9, 2005; Lueck, *Wall Street Journal*, February 9, 2005).

Now he tells us: former DHHS Secretary Tommy Thompson announced in his resignation speech that the new Medicare drug legislation should have allowed Medicare to negotiate directly with pharmaceutical companies for discounts on prescription drugs. The 2003 bill prohibits such bargaining. A *Boston Globe* editorial said the comments from Thompson "emphasize a major weakness" of the new law (Editorial, *Boston Globe*, December 8, 2004).

In a rare break with Big Pharma, the AMA adopted a policy in support of allowing the DHHS to negotiate with drug manufacturers for discounts on medications. The Medicare drug bill currently prohibits such bargaining. AMA officials noted that other federal agencies, such as the VA and Defense Department, are able to negotiate substantial cost savings (Pear, *New York Times*, October 17, 2004).

Only about one in five low-income Medicare beneficiaries who are eligible for a $600 drug subsidy have signed up for the benefit. James Firman, CEO of the National Council on the Aging, said that 5 million eligible seniors have not signed up because most "are confused and skeptical about the benefits" (Congressional Quarterly Healthbeat, December 6, 2004).

In an attempt to persuade seniors that the Medicare drug program is a good deal, the CMS is requiring Medigap insurers to send a notice to policy holders stating that the new drug benefit "will provide greater value than your current coverage." The National Association of Insurance Commissioners complained that the Bush administration was using "precisely the type of 'push' advertising that [insurance regulators] oppose and prohibit at the state regulatory level" (Pear, *New York Times*, November 7, 2004).

There is "insufficient evidence" to suggest that disease management programs would reduce Medicare spending, according to the Congressional Budget Office. The few studies reporting cost savings generally do not account for all health care costs, including the cost of the intervention itself. Although some evidence has indicated savings for programs designed for select groups of patients, little research exists that would be relevant to issues arising in the older and sicker Medicare population (Congressional Budget Office, "An Analysis of the Literature on Disease Management Programs," October 13, 2004).

POLLS AND PUBLIC OPINION

There is overwhelming support for providing government-funded health care to all children regardless of family income, according to a survey of 2,000 adults. The level of support for children's health care is similar to that for Medicare. Ninety percent of those surveyed said that government should fund health care for all low-income children and seniors, while almost the same percentage (84% for children, 87% for seniors) said such funding should be available regardless of family income (Berk et al., "Americans' Views about the Adequacy of Health Care for Children and the Elderly," *Health Affairs* Web Exclusive, September 14, 2004).

Forty-one percent of physicians supported single-payer in a 2004 poll by the AMA, up from 18 percent in 1992. Adopting single-payer national health insurance was more highly favored than expanding existing public programs to cover the uninsured (38%), an individual mandate to purchase coverage (27%), or an employer mandate (24%). By specialty, psychiatrists were the most likely to support single-payer (58%), while anesthesiologists were least likely to favor single-payer (30%). Interestingly, physicians over age 40 were more likely to favor single-payer (43%) than those under 40 (35%) (AMA Division of Market Research and Analysis, Advocacy Agenda Setting Survey, September 2004).

Two-thirds (66%) of U.S. residents say the cost of prescription drugs is "unreasonably high," according to a poll of 1,012 adults. Sixty percent of respondents favor government price controls on prescription drugs, and three-quarters (74%) cite marketing, advertising, or industry profits as the prime contributor to rising pharmaceutical prices. Only 22 percent cited research as the biggest contributor to rising drug costs (Harris Poll, "Prescription Drug Prices, Hospital Costs and Doctors' Fees," September 20, 2004).

Two-thirds (67%) of Americans say they support a health care "guarantee" like those provided by the governments of Canada and Great Britain, according to a national survey of 1,020 adults. About four-fifths say the U.S. government should regulate health care like utilities (78%) and negotiate bulk purchasing of prescription drugs to control costs (83%) (Civil Society Institute, "How Access and Affordability are Shaping Views," September 15, 2004).

Forty percent of U.S. residents believe that the quality of health care has worsened in the past five years, compared with 38 percent who believe it has stayed the same and 17 percent who believe it has improved. About 55 percent are dissatisfied with the quality of their own care, up from 44 percent five years ago. People with chronic conditions are more likely to express concern with the quality of care (66% to 53%) and to report having experienced a medical error in their own care or that of a family member (50% to 30%) (Agency for Health Care Quality and Research, "National Survey on Consumers' Experiences with Patient Safety Quality Information," November 17, 2004).

More than three-quarters of Americans have an unfavorable opinion of health savings accounts (HSAs) and similar high-deductible health plans (77%), and report they would feel vulnerable to high medical bills with this type of coverage (79%). Already, just 57 percent of insured adults under age 65 say they feel "well-protected" by their insurance plan, and many (38%) are worried that they will have unmet health care needs. HSA plans pair a tax-free health savings account with a high-deductible "catastrophic" policy (Kaiser Health Poll Report, September–October 2004.

A survey of 1,312 wealthy Americans who have at least $1 million to invest (not including the value of their home) indicates that wealth does not eliminate anxiety over increasing health care costs. A whopping 96 percent of millionaires under age 55 were "very worried" or "somewhat worried" that health costs would affect their retirement (Chu, *Wall Street Journal*, February 3, 2005).

INTERNATIONAL HEALTH SYSTEMS

In Canada, the federal government is committed to investing an additional $41.2 billion dollars in the Canadian health system over the next decade; $4.5 billion of the new federal funding is earmarked to reduce waiting times in five areas: cancer, heart, diagnostic imaging, joint replacements, and sight restoration (National Union, "A Full Evaluation of the 2004 First Ministers' 10-year Health Action Plan," September 2004).

The Canadian province of British Columbia will spend $5 million in 2005 to reduce waiting times for cardiac surgery. The province expects to boost the number of open-heart surgeries by 5 percent, and reduce the maximum waiting time to three months. British Columbia successfully reduced its waiting list by one-third over a ten-month period beginning in June 2003 with $3.4 million in extra funding and more effective recruitment of staff—especially critical care nurses. The number of people waiting for surgery decreased from 623 to 409 between June 2003 and April 2004. Median waiting times also dropped from 18 to 14.9 weeks. In the 2005 effort, $2 million is earmarked for high-risk patients (Jones, *Canadian Medical Association Journal*, September 14, 2004).

The U.S. infant mortality rate increased for the first time in 44 years in 2002, from 6.9 to 7.0 infants dying per 1,000 births. Compared with other nations, the U.S. ranks number 42 in infant mortality (Kristof, *New York Times*, January 12, 2005).

An estimated 150,000 foreigners traveled to India in 2003 to undergo medical procedures. A heart procedure that costs $200,000 in the United States is available for $10,000 in India. Although most "medical tourists" are from developing nations in Africa or the Middle East, at least one U.S. columnist has suggested that the United States send its uninsured to India for affordable health care (Lancaster, *Washington Post*, October 21, 2004).

Colombia serves as another popular "medical tourism" destination for Latin American immigrants living in the United States and those seeking significant savings from the cost of treatment in the American system. Colombia offers medical services at a fraction of the U.S. price, such as in vitro fertilization ($3,500 vs. $12,000 in the United States) and LASIK eye surgery ($510 per eye, vs. $1,814 in the United States). But many of the Colombian Americans who return home for care say the main draw is doctors who actually have the time to talk to their patients (Morris, *Florida Sun-Sentinel*, March 7, 2005).

The United States performs poorly on most measures of primary care, according to a study of 8,600 adults in five countries by the Commonwealth Fund. The United States ranked either last or near-last compared with Australia, Canada, New Zealand, and the United Kingdom on almost all dimensions of patient-centered care, including access, coordination, and physician-patient experiences. U.S. and Canadian adults are the least likely to see a doctor the same day when sick, and most likely to wait multiple days for care. U.S. patients are most likely to have high out-of-pocket costs and to forgo care because of costs. U.S. patients also reported the greatest difficulty in getting after-hours care.

While majorities of those surveyed in all nations report having a regular source of primary care, U.S. patients stood out for having shorter relationships with physicians, signaling a lack of care continuity. One-fourth of U.S. patients reported more than $1,000 in out-of-pocket medical costs in 2003, compared with 4 to 14 percent of patients in other countries. U.K. and Canadian patients had the lowest out-of-pocket costs.

Forty percent of U.S. patients went without care because of costs, compared with 10 to 33 percent in other nations. Although low-income adults were more likely to report access problems in all countries, only in the United States did a majority (57%) go without care due to costs (Canada, 14%; United Kingdom, 13%). U.S. residents were also the most likely (33%) to say their nation's health system needs to be "totally rebuilt" (Schoen et al., "Primary Care and Health System Performance: Adults' Experiences in Five Countries," *Health Affairs*, October 28, 2004).

HEALTH SAVINGS ACCOUNTS

Authors' note: Health savings accounts (HSAs; also called medical savings accounts, MSAs) are touted by the Bush administration as a "consumer-driven" solution to the health care crisis. HSAs, as noted above, combine a high-deductible health insurance plan (HDHP) with a tax-free savings account that can be used only for health expenses. The personal nature of the accounts means that sick people quickly exhaust their meager savings and face high out-of-pocket costs. Meanwhile, HSAs provide a tax subsidy to the healthy and wealthy. As the sickest 10 percent of the population uses 72 percent of health care, HSAs do nothing to lower costs. Money put into an HSA gets rolled over each year and can be withdrawn at retirement, removing the dollars of the healthy and wealthy from the insurance risk pool. The plans are very complex to administer, requiring the tracking of all out-of-pocket payments, and discourage prevention. Additionally, most HSA plans are PPOs, complete with the usual physician restrictions and cost-sharing.

More than 20 financial institutions are marketing HSAs, and 50 insurance companies have introduced the associated HDHP. HSAs, as defined by the new Medicare law, are available to people who purchase an HDHP with a deductible at or above $1,000 for an individual or $2,000 for a family, though family deductibles of $5,000 are not uncommon. Employees, employers, or both can contribute up to $2,600 for individuals or $5,150 for families. A recent study found that 81 percent of employers with 20,000 or more workers were either "somewhat" or "very" likely to offer HSAs by 2006 (*Wall Street Journal*, September 9, 2004; Kaiser, July 26, 2004).

California-based HMO Kaiser Permanente is starting to sell HDHPs in some markets. Kaiser officials said the company, which prides itself on its 60-year history of providing comprehensive coverage, is unable to compete with low-cost, bare-bones plans targeting the healthy. "If all we offer at Kaiser is comprehensive coverage, then all of the sick people go to Kaiser and everyone else goes to the other plans," said senior vice president Arthur Southam (Rundle, *Wall Street Journal*, November 15, 2004).

UnitedHealth Group, the nation's second largest health insurer, is positioning itself to capitalize on the growing demand for HDHPS and HSAs. UnitedHealth paid $800 million in 2004 for Golden Rule Financial, the family-owned firm that pioneered (and donated heavily to the Republican Party to pass) medical savings accounts. UnitedHealth pushed all its own employees into HDHPs this year. The Blue Cross Blue Shield Association announced that it will offer HSAs in 49 states by 2006 (Appleby, *USA Today*, October 9, 2003; Higgins, *Washington Times*, November 18, 2004).

One-third of hospitalized patients with deductibles of $1,000 would have paid more than 10 percent of their total income in out-of-pocket expenses in 2003 if they had the new HDHPs currently on the market, according to a study of projected cost-sharing scenarios of about 33,000 individuals. The HDHPs studied were similar to those currently being offered in combination with HSAs, including such features as 20 percent in-network coinsurance and 30 percent out-of-network coinsurance (Trude, "Patient Cost Sharing: How Much Is Too Much?" Center for Studying Health System Change, *Issue Brief* No. 72, December 2003).

High-deductible health plans often trick patients who are seeking relief from high premiums but who don't realize how poor the coverage may be. Many plans do not cover preventive care, and have high cost-sharing for covered services. Many also contain confusing rules that dictate what counts toward the deductible and what doesn't, such as only counting "reasonable and customary" charges by in-network providers against the deductible, rather than the actual amount paid. Many plans sharply limit benefits such as prescription drugs, rehabilitation, physical therapy, and mental health services, and out-of-pocket payments for these services do not count toward the deductible (Rubenstein, *Wall Street Journal*, January 28, 2005).

In a harbinger of what future HSA plans will look like, Blue Cross Blue Shield of North Carolina announced the introduction of its new HSA product. The plan combines an HDHP from Blue Cross with an HSA administered by Mellon Financial Corp. in the framework of a managed care PPO, with restricted provider lists and contracted fees. The same restrictions of the PPO apply to the HSA component of the coverage: patients that go to out-of-network providers will face financial penalties, and their out-of-pocket costs will not apply to the plan's deductible (Blue Cross Blue Shield of North Carolina, press release, December 2, 2004).

Note—This article is adapted from a report published by Physicians for a National Health Program in the *PNHP Newsletter,* Summer 2005.

Reproduced with kind permission of *International Journal of Health Services,* (Volume 36, Number 1, Pages 157–176, 2006)

Direct reprint requests to:

Nicholas Skala

Physicians for a National Health Program 29 East Madison Street, Suite 602

Chicago, IL 60602

e-mail: nick@pnhp.org

Declaration of Thessaloniki Conference

This XIVth Conference of the IAHPE began with a reminder of the importance of the Hippocratic, humanist values that are under constant attack from the growing tendency towards market-style reforms and privatisation in health care systems.

This conference condemns the way in which governments and those directing health care across Europe are using the people of East and West Europe as guinea-pigs in a grotesque experiment in the use of untested market mechanisms in place of any planned allocation of health care resources, or any reference to principles of equity and social solidarity.

Conference further notes the lack of any systematic evidence to support these reforms or process of evaluation of their impact where they have been implemented. We reject the notion that greater use of private sector providers either reduces costs of improves efficiency, and note that this approach works strongly against equity and social solidarity.

This conference condemns the way in which the agenda at EU and national level is increasingly shaped around easing the level of regulation to favour the commercial interests of the pharmaceutical companies. These corporations rush to exploit profitable markets for new patented drugs, while their research programmes largely ignore the burden of preventable disease and some of the major health care problems affecting the world's poor and disadvantaged.

Conference has noted the consequences of this line of policy:

● In Germany, charges have been imposed for visiting a doctor, aimed at reducing the numbers accessing health care;

● In the United Kingdom, a huge expansion of government spending on private provision of care for National Health Service patients threatens to destabilise the public sector provision in many areas

● In Turkey, the privatisation of hospital services has run alongside a growing inequality in access to health care

● Greece has emerged as the country in which the highest share of total health spending comes from private "out of pocket" payments, while public spending on health at just over 2% of GDP is one of the lowest in Europe.

● In Palestine, the drive to increased reliance on private for profit treatment is driven by the active policy of donor organisations

● In many European countries and around the world, co-payments or user fees are being imposed on health treatment, designed to reduce demand, and press more people towards private insurance cover.

This Conference rejects these policies as detrimental to the health needs of the people of Europe. We call instead for a new initiative that will link up campaigners, academics, health professionals, trade unionists and progressive social movements that will seek to:

■ Expose the real content of the policies and so-called "reforms" based on neoliberalism, privatisation and marketisation

■ Challenge governments and political leaders to examine, discuss and debate the impact of these policies and the possibility of a very different approach based on principles of multi-disciplinary cooperation, equity, and social solidarity

■ Pursue the campaign for the strict regulation and control of the pharmaceutical corporations, and the establishment of health care systems that are universal, democratically controlled and accountable to local people, responsive to service users, supportive to health care staff, publicly and equitably funded, and delivered free to all at point of use.

IAHPE
Thessaloniki, May 29 2005

Contributors to this volume

Gunnar Ågren,
> Director General, Swedish National Institute of Public Health, Stockholm, Sweden

Feride Aksu Sacaklioglu
> Public Health, Ege University, Turkey

Lila Antonopoulou
> Associate Professor, Department of Economics, Aristotle University of Thessaloniki, Greece

Fatih Artvinli
> People's Health Movement, Istanbul, Turkey

Alexis Benos
> Social Medicine, Aristotle University, Thessaloniki, Greece

Hans Ulrich Deppe
> Institut für Medizinische Soziologie, Fachbereich Medizin Johann Wolfgang Goethe-Universität Frankfurt Frankfurt a.M. Germany

Tim Dodd
> Medical Faculty, University of Kragujevac, Kragujevac, Serbia

Aleksandar Dzakula
> Andrija Stampar School of Public Health, Medical School, Zagreb, Croatia

Magda Gavana
> Social Medicine, Aristotle University, Thessaloniki, Greece

Thomas Gerlinger
> Institut für Medizinische Soziologie, Fachbereich Medizin Johann Wolfgang Goethe-Universität Frankfurt Frankfurt a.M. Germany

Stathis Giannakopoulos
Social Medicine, Aristotle University, Thessaloniki, Greece
Motasem Hamdan Ph.D.
Health Policy and Management Unit, School of Public Health, Al-Quds University, Palestine
Onur Hamzaoglu
Public Health, Kocaeli University, Turkey
Ida Hellander
Physicians for a National Health Programme (PNHP), USA
Slobodan Jankovic
Medical Faculty, University of Kragujevac, Kragujevac, Serbia
Mauri Johansson
Public Health Partner, Specialist in Community & Occupational Medicine, Bording, Denmark
J.Karadzinska -Bislimovska
Institute of Occupational Health, WHO Collaborating Center for Occupational Health, Skopje, Macedonia
Elias Kondilis
Social Medicine, Aristotle University, Thessaloniki, Greece
Jane Lethbridge
Public Services International Research Unit (PSIRU)
The Business School, University of Greenwich, London, UK
John Lister
Information Director, London Health Emergency, UK
Associate Senior Lecturer, Coventry University, UK
Philip van Meurs
Political Scientist, Brussels, Belgium
Jadranka Mustajbegovic
Andrija Stampar School of Public Health, Medical School, Zagreb, Croatia

Susanne Öhrling
Swedish National Institute of Public Health, Stockholm, Sweden

Nikolina Radakovic, MD
Andrija Stampar School of Public Health, Medical School, Zagreb, Croatia

S.Risteska-Kuc
Institute of Occupational Health, WHO Collaborating Center for Occupational Health, Skopje, Macedonia

Rolf Rosenbrock
Wissenschaftszentrum Berlin für Sozialforschung (WZB)
Social Science Research Center Berlin
AG Public Health Research Unit, Public Health Policy
Berlin, Germany

Rolf Schmucker
Institut für Medizinische Soziologie
Fachbereich Medizin   Goethe-Universität Frankfurt, Germany

Nicholas Skala
Physicians for a National Health Programme (PNHP), USA

Luka Voncina, MSc, MD
Andrija Stampar School of Public Health, Medical School, Zagreb, Croatia

Theodore Zdoukos
Social Medicine, Aristotle University, Thessaloniki, Greece

driving societies backward
Critical analysis of the dominant health policies
ongoing neoliberal reform
Declaration rejects the policies as detrimental
to the health needs of the people of Europe.
.Slow transformation of health care into a commodity
194 features of public service provision are abrogated (Turkey
195
197 This is a regression in terms of social right

Printed in the United Kingdom
by Lightning Source UK Ltd.
124688UK00001B/46-72/A

9 780955 733307